The questions of how to define futile treatments and how to find agreement among the various stakeholders in decisions about life-sustaining interventions are among the most challenging in medical practice. This book surveys the clinical, ethical, religious, legal, economic, and personal dimensions of decision making in situations where the choice is between extending costly medical treatment of uncertain effectiveness and terminating treatment, thereby ending the patient's life.

Contributors from a wide range of disciplines offer perspectives on issues ranging from the definition of medical futility to the implications for care in various clinical settings, including intensive care, neonatal and pediatric practice, and nursing homes. Notable legal cases are examined, including many that have helped to define the issues and move forward the debate, and there is powerful testimony from the point of view of families of patients in futile treatment situations.

Although a consensus on what constitutes futile treatment remains elusive, the eloquence and concern manifested in this book, and its critical analysis of positions that are frequently conflicting, will certainly contribute in a large way toward the more humane and consistent handling of these situations. *Medical Futility* will be obligatory reading for health care professionals, students, and scholars concerned with ethical standards in medical care.

MEDICAL FUTILITY

MEDICAL FUTILITY

and the evaluation of life-sustaining interventions

Edited by

MARJORIE B. ZUCKER

Choice In Dying
New York

HOWARD D. ZUCKER

The Mount Sinai School of Medicine
New York

Foreword by Alexander Morgan Capron
University of Southern California
Los Angeles

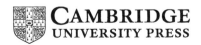

CAMBRIDGE
UNIVERSITY PRESS

PUBLISHED BY THE PRESS SYNDICATE OF THE UNIVERSITY OF CAMBRIDGE
The Pitt Building, Trumpington Street, Cambridge CB2 1RP, United Kingdom

CAMBRIDGE UNIVERSITY PRESS
The Edinburgh Building, Cambridge CB2 2RU, United Kingdom
40 West 20th Street, New York, NY 10011-4211, USA
10 Stamford Road, Oakleigh, Melbourne 3166, Australia

First published 1997

Printed in the United States of America

Typeset in Times Roman

Library of Congress Cataloging-in-Publication Data
Medical futility : and the evaluation of life-sustaining interventions
/ edited by Marjorie B. Zucker, Howard D. Zucker.
p.   cm.
Includes index.
ISBN 0-521-56020-9 (hc). – ISBN 0-521-56877-3 (pb)
1. Terminal care.   2. Medical ethics.   I. Zucker, Marjorie B.
(Marjorie Bass), 1919–   .   II. Zucker, Howard David.
R726.M36   1997
362.1'75 – dc20   96–46070
                                                        CIP

A catalog record for this book is available from
the British Library

ISBN 0-521-56020-9 hardback
ISBN 0-521-56877-3 paperback

Contents

Preface

One of us (M.B.Z.), a retired bench scientist via a medical family, has had a long commitment to Choice In Dying, a national not-for-profit organization dedicated to fostering communication about complex end-of-life decisions among individuals, their loved ones, and health care professionals. The organization is well known for inventing living wills in 1967 and providing the only national hotline to respond to patients and families during end-of-life crises. Choice In Dying also provides award-winning educational materials, public and physician education, and ongoing monitoring of changes in state and federal right-to-die legislation.

The other (H.D.Z.), in addition to sharing his spouse's interests, was in medical practice before becoming a consultation-liaison psychiatrist. He thus has had practical experience with dying patients as well as in teaching medical students and residents at the Mount Sinai Medical Center. When the opportunity arose to edit a book on medical futility, it seemed natural to do so as coeditors.

We are obligated to all who contributed chapters for taking on the task in the midst of their very busy lives and for their flexibility in accepting suggestions and making revisions. We hope that the resulting book proves timely and stimulating to readers of all ages and many disciplines and that it helps introduce younger readers to some of the issues relating to end-of-life care.

We are pleased to acknowledge another collaboration: the production of four children and our enjoyment of them and of our four children-in-law, and our eight grandchildren.

Marjorie B. Zucker, Ph.D.
Howard D. Zucker, M.D.

Foreword

ALEXANDER MORGAN CAPRON, LL.B.

University Professor of Law and Medicine,
University of Southern California, Los Angeles

Many aspects of modern medicine provoke spirited ethical argument, but few engender as much disagreement about what exactly is at issue as does the futility debate. The relationships of physicians and nurses, on the one side, and patients (especially dying patients dependent on extensive medical support) and their families, on the other, are viewed very differently by various commentators. As characterized by some, physicians have become pathetic characters in a modern day Molière play, technically sophisticated servants doing the bidding of their patients. Professionals with this perception feel misused and justify their rebelliousness by invoking medical futility. The simple recognition of the limits of medicine's power to cure and to extend life denotes that health care professionals should not be obliged to provide further treatment or, more powerfully, that they would exceed their role-based authority as healers to continue to do so. Yet other commentators claim that medical futility is an empty concept that does not provide any ground for decision that would not be present had the concept never been coined. They characterize medical futility as nothing more than a cover for physician's rearguard action to regain the dominance in decision making that they possessed before autonomy and informed consent shifted authority to patients and their families beginning in the 1960s.

Although much of the futility debate of recent years has been premised on the notion that one ought to pick among these (and many other) sharply contrasting conceptions, each advocated with great conviction, it may be just as reasonable to regard these different descriptions as distinct facets of the larger whole of medical futility. If medical futility is likened to the fabled elephant, these various commentators are the blind men, each describing the beast differently because each feels a different part of its anatomy.

Why all this concern about medical futility? Three factors may account for its emergence as the subject of lively debate. The first is the nature of

medicine as practiced in the United States in the second half of the twentieth
century. Fed by an ever increasing array of life-sustaining technologies –
most notably, those connected with cardiopulmonary resuscitation (CPR) and
those that constitute the foundation of the intensive care unit (ICU) – medicine has not only extended the lives of many critically ill patients and
changed the way people die but also made it necessary to make choices about
when to use and when to forgo these powerful but imperfect interventions.
Disputes about how and by whom these choices should be made provoked
heated debate within health care institutions that, in the 1970s, became increasingly public. Typically, such disagreements pitted a patient, such as
Elizabeth Bouvia, or a family, such as the parents of Karen Ann Quinlan,
who wanted to discontinue treatment, against physicians and others who insisted that the resulting death would be wrong morally, professionally, and
legally. By 1990, when the United States Supreme Court addressed the issue
in its landmark *Cruzan* decision, it was generally agreed that a decision to
forgo treatment – whether made by a patient contemporaneously or through
an advance directive, or by a surrogate legally authorized to act on the patient's behalf – ought usually to be respected, even when stopping (or not
starting) the treatment would probably result in the patient's death. The existence of a broad consensus on this point has not, however, removed the
need for choices to be made, nor has it eliminated all disputes. Health care
providers and patients (and families) continue to disagree in some cases about
whether it is appropriate to forgo treatment. Today, however, in the most
contentious cases, the roles are reversed from the pattern of the 1970s and
1980s, with patients and families now insisting on further interventions, and
physicians and others in health care wanting to stop.

The second factor driving the medical futility debate is the current reexamination of the principle of autonomy. Not just in the end-of-life context
but more generally, the dominance of this principle is being challenged both
in bioethics theory and in the policies and rules that guide health care. Are
there not times when the claims of the community outweigh individual preferences? Or when a decision cannot be left solely to the patient but must
bow to the conscience of the physician or other health care provider in practicing his or her profession? One reason that the futility debate engenders
such heated exchanges is precisely because, on the one hand, some physicians
believe that yielding to the wishes of patients and, even more so, next-of-kin
that futile treatment be continued is an abdication of their role as medical
professionals. They argue that, consistent with the goals of medicine since
the time of Hippocrates, physicians not only have no obligation to treat – or
even to present such options to patients and families – when medical inter-

ventions cannot produce a sufficient quality of life (such as restoring consciousness and the ability to live without continuous life support) but also that physicians cease behaving professionally if they persist even when no medically valid goal remains. On the other hand, advocates for patient rights see this position as simply a new instance of medical paternalism. Even those who would admit that the pendulum of decision-making authority may have swung too far in the direction of patient autonomy are worried that accepting the concept of medical futility would propel the pendulum back to the side of expert domination of health care decisions. In their view, questions of quality of life are inherently personal, not technical, and hence provide no ground for physicians or other professionals to impose their ideas of what constitutes an outcome of sufficient value to justify further treatment.

Although these two factors – the choices that modern medicine generates about end-of-life care and the reexamination of the meaning of autonomy in medical decision making – would be enough to ensure medical futility a prominent place in bioethics discussions and an occasional court case, a third force accounts for futility's becoming a conspicuous part of the broader public debates over health care. That force is the emergence of managed care as the dominant mode of health care delivery in this country. Like a tidal wave, managed care is sweeping aside old ways of providing care, reconfiguring the relationships of physicians, hospitals, insurers, payers, and the insured population. The explanation for this rapid transformation lies not in any wish of providers to reorganize themselves nor even in the understandable desire of employers and insurers to shift some of the risk of escalating health care costs onto other shoulders. The real attraction of managed care, to corporate payers as well as to public policymakers and perhaps even to individuals, is its promise to reduce health care expenditures by eliminating nonbeneficial interventions. Whether or not the skeptics are right that the impressive results of some managed care programs are just one-time savings achieved by forcing physicians and hospitals to discount their prices without halting the upward spiral that comes from new medical technologies and an aging population, it is generally agreed that eliminating truly useless medical interventions will not be enough. Some care that might provide benefit (yet at a low probability) or that will provide marginal benefit (yet at great cost) must also be eliminated if managed care or any other system is to succeed in controlling health care expenditures.

Particularly in the context of critically ill, dying patients, the provision of care that cannot reverse their decline might well be described as a futile effort. Thus, the terminology that has emerged in the current debates, that medical futility has both a quantitative dimension (when the probability of getting the desired result is very small) and a qualitative one (when the best projected outcome would not truly benefit the patient), not only fits into managed care's paradigm of limiting marginal care but actually provides what for such commentators as Daniel Callahan and Richard Lamm seems a particularly compelling illustration of the wisdom of imposing such limits: at the end of a long life, patients should not seek, and society should not provide, treatments aimed at holding off the natural process of degeneration but should instead seek to make their dying an integrated and accepted part of living. Better, they claim, that health care dollars be spent where, on average, they have a better chance to provide true benefits than to pour the large percentage we now do into the final days and weeks of life. Of course, such a position has yet to be adopted by most Americans, philosophically or emotionally, and decisions defended on the grounds of futility are likely to be resisted by the individuals who would thus be denied care and to become rallying points in the judicial and legislative arenas for advocates objecting to the goals or the means of the managed care firms and politicians who are trying to limit patients' access to the full range of medical interventions.

This book is intended both to clarify the questions at issue in the futility debate and to move beyond the theoretical contours of that debate and illuminate how decisions about care are and ought to be made in a variety of settings and with a variety of patients. Currently, much of the discussion of futility has focused on acute care settings, such as ICUs and emergency rooms, and on emergency interventions, such as CPR. Although the book opens by attending to these issues, subsequent chapters explore general medical, pediatric, and nursing home care and the influence of ethnicity and related factors on patients' and physicians' views of what it means to give up on medical care. The authors then address the cultural, religious, and psychologic influences in conflicts about futility as well as the economic aspects of limiting treatment that has been labeled ''futile.'' Next, the book examines the roles of ethics committees, the courts, the professions, the community, and health care institutions in setting standards for, and helping to resolve disputes about, decisions at the end of life. The volume closes with warnings about some of the significant risks related to medical futility: abuse of vulnerable populations, a return to medical dominance, decision making either polarized in courtroom confrontations or sent askew by misguided institutional policies, and clinical and financial pressures that may override patients' best interests.

Readers need not despair, however, for this volume will enrich their understanding of health care decision making and provide rays of hope that greater attention will result in more research on the definition of futile care and the consequences of limiting it, and that the open development of policies and procedures for limiting care of marginal benefit can avoid arbitrary instances of forgoing treatment or even withholding information from patients when physicians feel incapable of producing results they judge to be beneficial. The clinically and theoretically diverse contributions to this volume provide an excellent starting point for all those who wish to get past the rhetoric of the futility debate. With our blindfolds removed, we can appreciate the separate parts of the medical futility elephant as manifestations of something that is complicated rather than contradictory and, with luck, arrive at an understanding of the subject in all its rich complexity.

Contributors

Ellen Knapik Bartoldus, M.S.W.
Assistant Administrator, Wartburg Lutheran Home for the Aging, Brooklyn, NY

Howard Brody, M.D., Ph.D.
Professor of Family Practice and Philosophy and Director, Center for Ethics and Humanities in the Life Sciences, Michigan State University, East Lansing, MI

Patricia Brophy, R.N.
South Easton, MA

Sarah Gelbach DeMichele, M.D.
Assistant Instructor of Psychiatry, University of Pennsylvania, Philadelphia, PA

Martin Drooker, M.D.
Assistant Clinical Professor of Psychiatry and Associate Director of the Psychiatric Consultation Service, The Mount Sinai Medical Center, New York, NY

Joel E. Frader, M.D.
Associate Professor of Pediatrics and of Anesthesiology and Critical Care Medicine and Associate Director, Center for Medical Ethics, University of Pittsburgh, Pittsburgh, PA

Alice Herb, J.D., LL.M.
Assistant Clinical Professor, Humanities in Medicine, SUNY Health Science Center, Brooklyn, NY

Joseph J. Jacobs, M.D., M.B.A.,
First Director, Office of Alternative Medicine, National Institutes of Health, Bethesda, MD (Present address, Guilford, CT)

Linda Johnson, M.S.W.
Project Facilitator, Midwest Bioethics Center, Kansas City, MO

Karen Orloff Kaplan, M.P.H., Sc.D.
Executive Director, Choice In Dying, New York, NY

Eliot J. Lazar, M.D.
Chairman, Department of Medicine, The Brooklyn Hospital Center, and Associate Professor of Clinical Medicine, New York University School of Medicine, New York, NY

Anna Moretti, R.N., J.D.
Formerly Director of Program and Legal Services, Choice In Dying, New York, NY

Mary F. Morrison, M.D.
Assistant Professor of Psychiatry and Medicine, University of Pennsylvania, Philadelphia, PA

Donald J. Murphy, M.D.
Regional Medical Director, GeriMed of America, Inc., and Director, Colorado Collective for Medical Decisions, Inc., Denver, CO

John J. Paris, S.J., Ph.D.
Walsh Professor of Bioethics, Boston College, Chestnut Hill, MA, and Clinical Professor of Family Medicine and Community Health, Tufts University School of Medicine, Boston, MA

Mark Poorman, C.S.C., Ph.D.
Assistant Professor of Theology, University of Notre Dame, Notre Dame, IN

Robert Lyman Potter, M.D., Ph.D.
Clinical Ethics Scholar, Midwest Bioethics Center, Kansas City, MO

William Prip, M.A.
Formerly Program Associate for Legislative Affairs, Choice In Dying, New York, NY

Harry S. Rafkin, M.D.
Pittsburgh Critical Care Associates, St. Francis Medical Center, Pittsburgh, PA

Thomas Rainey, M.D.
Fellow, College of Critical Care Medicine; Director, Critical Care, Fairfax Hospital; President and CEO, Critical Med, Inc.; Adjunct Associate Professor of Anesthesia, George Washington University of Health Sciences; and Associate Clinical Professor of Internal Medicine, Georgetown University Hospital, Washington, DC

Stephen L. Snyder, M.D.
Assistant Clinical Professor of Psychiatry and Director of the Psychiatric Consultation Service, The Mount Sinai Medical Center, New York, NY

Bethany Spielman, Ph.D., J.D.
Assistant Professor of Medical Humanities, Southern Illinois University School of Medicine, Springfield, IL, and Assistant Professor of Medical Jurisprudence, Southern Illinois University School of Law, Carbondale, IL

Norton Spritz, M.D., J.D.
Chief, Medical Service, Department of Veterans Affairs Medical Center, and Professor of Medicine, New York University School of Medicine, New York, NY

James J. Strain, M.D.
Professor of Psychiatry and Director, Division of Behavioral Medicine and Consultation Psychiatry, The Mount Sinai Medical Center, New York, NY

Jon Watchko, M.D.
Associate Professor of Pediatrics, Obstetrics, Gynecology and Reproductive Services, University of Pittsburgh School of Medicine, and Department of Pediatrics, Magee-Womens Hospital, Pittsburgh, PA

1

Medical futility: a useful concept?

HOWARD BRODY, M.D., PH.D.

The problem of medical futility involves two questions.

1. Are there medical interventions in a specific patient with a particular disease that we can label *futile* or *useless* because we are sufficiently confident that they will not be beneficial?
2. If so, are physicians entitled, or indeed obligated, to refuse to provide those interventions to the patient in question even if the treatment is requested or demanded by the patient or appropriate surrogate?

Those who argue that futility is a dangerous or unhelpful concept that should be abandoned rest their case on the observation that these two questions are extremely hard to answer. I agree that attempting to answer these questions leads us into a thicket of a peculiarly vexing nature, the like of which has seldom been encountered in medical ethics. However, I argue that the concept of futility is unavoidable or can be avoided only by paying far too high a price. We have no choice but to enter the thicket and seek whatever compasses and machetes will best allow us to navigate.

In this chapter, I review some of the arguments commonly raised against the concept of medical futility and then indicate why I think that futility judgments are unavoidable nonetheless. Next, I argue that futility is so closely bound up with critical concepts of professional integrity that medicine risks losing its moral bearings if it ignores the issue. Finally, I suggest that arguments that seem perplexing in the abstract are more resolvable at the level of practical policy. Thus, it may be at the practical level – particularly by asking what sorts of discussions we want to take place within health care institutions – that we will eventually come to understand what futility means and what its appropriate limitations are.

Anti-futility arguments

Bernard Lo (1995) has carefully reviewed arguments against permitting physicians to make unilateral futility judgments. Lo argues for a moderate position – that futility judgments can sometimes be justified but that the concept is "fraught with confusion, inconsistency, and controversy" (1995:73). However, the arguments that he reviews have been used by more skeptical authors as reasons to dispense entirely with the concept of futility in medical ethics. Hence, for our purposes, Lo's list of concerns summarizes the anti-futility position.

Lo starts by granting that there are some senses of the word "futility" that appear to justify a unilateral decision to withhold a treatment. These include the following: the treatment has no pathophysiologic rationale, the patient is not responding even when treatment is at its maximal level, the treatment has already been given to the patient and the patient has not responded, and it is nearly certain that the treatment will not achieve the goals that the patient has specified. (An example of the fourth category might be the patient's stated desire to leave the hospital to return home, whereas the treatment would only succeed, at best, in keeping the patient alive in the intensive care unit dependent on machines.)

Lo distinguishes these more legitimate senses of futility from other commonly encountered usages of the term today: the likelihood of success is very small but not zero, the goals that the physicians perceive to be worthwhile cannot be achieved, the patient's quality of life is unacceptable, and the prospective benefit is not worth the resources required. It is easy to find examples of futility being used in each of Lo's questionable senses, both in the hallways of hospitals and even in the medical literature. This highlights Lo's point that the term may simply be too slippery to be allowed into the vocabulary of ethical discourse.

Besides this inconsistency in the use of the term "futility," Lo sees other problems with the concept. Futility judgments may be mistaken. We lack precise data on the usefulness of common treatments for many conditions, and it is easy for physicians to confuse either their frustration that the patient is not responding better to treatment or their distaste for the patient's present quality of life with scientific assessments of the likelihood of improvement. This leads directly to Lo's next problem: value judgments may be mistaken for factual or scientific expertise. It has become commonplace in today's medical ethics to distinguish between issues of technical knowledge, in which the physician legitimately claims expertise, and questions of value, in which physicians are duty bound to respect the wishes of the autonomous patient. With that model, unilateral physician futility judgments can easily slide into what Robert Veatch (1973) called "generalization of expertise," with physicians illegitimately claiming authority over the value judgments that patients ought to be allowed to make. Lo adds that one may not need to employ the specific language of futility to commit this ethical error. For instance, a decision that a treatment is "not medically indicated" may mask an illegitimate value judgment.

After reading Lo's list of concerns, many would conclude that medical ethics would be much better off without any appeals to futility (just as many have tried to eliminate appeals to the distinction between ordinary and extraordinary care as being more likely to mislead than to illuminate). The anti-futility camp fears that futility judgments may turn the clock back to the bad old days of physician paternalism by granting physicians unilateral powers to make treatment decisions. Moreover, the slipperiness of the concept assures us that if we allow physicians to make such decisions in the clearest cases, they will easily slide into making unjustified decisions in the muddier cases. To borrow a concept from Jay Katz (1984), we have been trying during the modern era of medical ethics to encourage a special sort of conversation between physician and patient, which invites the patient to become an active, informed participant in therapeutic decisions. Now, the futility supporters would replace conversation with silence, as physicians conclude that they can resolve these knotty questions without discussing the issues with patients or families.

The nature of the debate is further illustrated by one specific definitional dispute. Schneiderman and Jecker (1995) have suggested that a treatment should be considered futile when it has not worked once in the last 100 times it was tried. Waisel and Truog (1995) attack this definition by noting that the criterion is statistically equivalent to saying that a therapy is futile if physicians are 95% confident that it would be successful no more than 3 in 100 – a mathematical truism that Schneiderman et al. (1990) had themselves admitted in an earlier publication. Waisel and Truog find this an unacceptably loose definition and argue instead for a definition of strict physiologic futility – that is, a treatment is futile only when it is unable to achieve its physiologic objective. Cardiopulmonary resuscitation (CPR), for instance, would be futile if it failed to restore heartbeat and circulation but not if it kept the patient alive for an hour before suffering a second cardiac arrest and dying. Although these authors believe that their physiologic definition is superior because it avoids controversial value judgments, in fact it makes a value judgment that physicians ought to find especially controversial – that when we administer therapy, we care only what happens to the organs, and we do not care what happens to the patient.

CPR: are futility judgments avoidable in practice?

No matter how powerful the arguments for throwing the term "futility" out of the lexicon may seem, they fail if it can be shown that physicians must make value-laden futility judgments whether they like it or not. To make the case that this is so, I take a somewhat lengthy detour into the practice of CPR in hospitals.

It is standard practice in U.S. hospitals and emergency care settings to attempt CPR if a patient is discovered without pulse or respiration from a recent cardiac arrest. CPR was developed in the early 1960s to address a new opportunity for intervention – the coronary care unit with electronic monitoring of otherwise healthy patients who had recently sustained serious heart damage. This new setting allowed for the concentration of highly trained personnel near the patient's bedside and instantaneous notification of the onset of a potentially fatal rhythm disturbance of the heart. In this setting, CPR soon was shown to be successful about 50% of the time. Later, similar success rates were shown when CPR was used in patients with drug overdoses and in patients who suffered cardiac arrest or arrhythmias during general anesthesia.

The success of CPR led to a phenomenon fairly typical of American medicine – the uncritical use of technology that has proved beneficial to a small number of patients for treating other patients who have not been shown to benefit. CPR soon became the standard reaction to any patient in any U.S. health care setting who suffered a cardiac arrest. It was not until the late 1980s that research showed that although CPR still had about a 50% success rate in the populations of patients for whom it was initially designed, its success rate rapidly fell to 20% or less when it was applied to patients in other settings. There were even subpopulations in which the success rate was so close to zero that the label "futile" seemed appropriate. In general terms, CPR seems uniformly to be unsuccessful in patients who suffer a cardiac arrest in the face of concomitant failure of one or more major organ systems, overwhelming infection, or metastatic cancer (Moss 1989).

The debate over futility has focused on the decision to write a "do not attempt resuscitation" (DNAR)[1] order in the patient's chart. If this order

---

[1] A common but less precise usage is do not resuscitate (DNR). All the other authors in this volume use DNR rather than DNAR.

appears, CPR will not be performed if a serious arrhythmia or cardiac arrest occurs. If no such order appears, in the event of an arrest, a CPR team applies a combination of external chest compression, mechanical ventilation by mask or endotracheal tube, cardiac drugs, and electroshock according to well-recognized protocols. Heartbeat may be restored within 5 or 10 minutes, but, more commonly, after about 30 minutes of intense effort – perhaps 45 or even 60 minutes if the patient is young or previously healthy – the physician in charge of the team will decide that further efforts are pointless, and the code will be terminated.

The pro-futility side argues that in situations in which CPR is predictably without benefit (because of near zero success rates in scientific studies) and the patient or family will not agree to a DNAR order despite full explanations of these facts, physicians should be empowered to enter a DNAR order uni-laterally. The rebuttal from the anti-futility side is that any decision to enter a DNAR order is fraught with value-laden assumptions – what counts as a benefit and what counts as sufficient evidence of lack of benefit, to mention just two. According to this line of argument, physicians can never ethically impose their values on patients without patients' consent, especially when life and death may hang in the balance.

I have gone into this much detail about CPR to make one critically im-portant point. To my knowledge, all of the discussion about unilateral deci-sion making, value judgments, and futility relates to the decision whether or not to start CPR. I am aware of no serious policy consideration ever being given to demanding the consent of the patient or family as to when to stop CPR. In principle, however, these two decisions seem equally value laden. After all, no one can say with total certainty that the patient could not have responded if a code that was stopped at 45 minutes had continued for another 15 minutes, or that the extra 15 minutes of effort might not have provided some benefit (even if only psychologic comfort) to some party in the case. No one on the anti-futility side of the debate, however, seems upset that physicians are allowed to make reasonable judgments about what is working or not working and unilaterally decide to stop the code based on those judg-ments.

The reason it does not bother them and does not bother the vast majority of patients and families is obvious – when one considers all aspects of the practical situation, no other policy makes any sense. This feature of how CPR decisions are made in the real world illustrates conclusively to me that those on the anti-futility side of the debate are caught in a logical contradic-tion. If they are so worried about unilateral physician decision making whether to start CPR, they should be equally worried about unilateral physician decision making when to stop CPR. If they are not, I allege that they must be confused. I suggest that they cannot logically defend a patient's right to demand CPR when the patient is 87 and has widely metastatic cancer and pneumonia yet fail to defend the right of a patient or family to demand that the code team continue CPR for at least 12 hours.

Although I have claimed that the anti-futility position ultimately cannot succeed, the strong arguments raised by Lo and others ought to cause us considerable unease when we contemplate physicians who misuse the futility concept or refuse to discuss critical decisions with patients. I argue that we should take those concerns very seriously but that we can do so within a framework that admits the occasional justification for physician determination of futility. However, we first have to be very clear on what ethical concerns are at stake in physician futility judgments. This, in turn, forces us to undertake a discussion of professional integrity. Furthermore, we must address practical policy matters to ensure that appeals to futility and to physician integrity are used to start and not to stop useful conversations between physicians and patients.

Futility and professional integrity

The ethical principle of patient autonomy seems to require that value-laden medical decisions be discussed with the patient and that the patient be allowed the last word. If, in futility cases, the physician's determination is supposed to carry more weight than the patient's own choice, we need to appeal to some countervailing ethical principle to explain why. I propose that the relevant principle is respect for professional integrity (Brody 1994).

The principle of professional integrity has been (sadly) little discussed in recent work on medical ethics, compared with such principles as autonomy, beneficence, and justice. This chapter is not the place for an extended analysis, but a few critical points can be offered.

Professional integrity appears as an ethical principle if we start with the assumption that medical practice has some sort of core moral content and that physicians make a moral commitment of some sort when they profess to practice medicine. As Pellegrino and Thomasma (1981) have argued, medicine is not defined either as a science or as an application of science. Instead, it is best understood as the application of scientific principles to individual cases with the goal of promoting a right and good healing action. Therefore, at least some ethical standards are defined by the nature of the practice of medicine itself, and physicians of integrity are required to adhere to those standards.

Consider some commonplace examples of things we typically expect of physicians of integrity.

1. Not to perform surgery for people who do not have the disease for which the surgery is usually indicated
2. Not to prescribe anabolic steroids for teenage body-builders
3. Not to engage in sexual relationships with their patients

Notice two important things about this list. First, we do not specify anything about the patient's level of autonomy or information. We do not, for example, say that if the teenage bodybuilder has exhaustively read all available scientific articles on the benefits and risks of anabolic steroids, it would be all right to prescribe them. We assume that since the appeal here is to the standards that define medicine as a type of practice, physicians as a group have legitimate say over those standards, even though physicians do not practice in a social vacuum and even if professional–public dialogue and negotiation are ultimately critical in formulating ethically defensible standards.

Second, this list is independent of the physician's personal value system. Consider two physicians, one with religious views strongly opposing sterilization, the second with different philosophical views. If the first physician were to perform sterilizations, we would hold that he lacked personal integrity because one crucial aspect of his behavior stood opposed to values that he claimed to be important in defining his moral identity. We would not say this of the second physician were he to perform sterilizations. We would hold, however, that both physicians were equally lacking in professional integrity if they prescribed anabolic steroids or surgically removed gallbladders known in advance to be healthy.

It is important to see that medicine may have internal ethical standards that define its legitimate practice, even when these standards are subject to heated controversy. Consider the debate over physician-assisted suicide and euthanasia. Some argue that these actions would be permissible for physicians in extreme cases, as when a competent patient was suffering terribly and had no other available means to relieve suffering. Others would argue that such actions are contrary to the internal moral standards of physicians, who should always strive to be healers and never to be agents of death. Some would conclude from the vigorous and unresolved debate over this question that medicine cannot have any internal, defining ethical standards, or we would expect near unanimity on such a critical issue. I claim instead that this debate shows that it makes good sense to talk about internal ethical standards because there would be no point to the debate if medicine did not have such standards.

What does this have to do with futility? The example of unnecessary surgery suggests that physician integrity includes an injunction not to perform actions that predictably fail to offer benefit (and that could, in some cases, cause harm). With a more detailed analysis of the elements of professional integrity (Miller and Brody 1995), the following reasons emerge.

1. The ethical goals that define medical practice include healing and curing disease, promoting health and preventing disease, and relieving suffering caused by disease symptoms. If a treatment can be reasonably predicted not to do any of these, to require that physicians offer it is to require them to act contrary to their goals of practice.
2. Physicians are obligated to adhere to high standards of scientific competence. Employing a treatment that predictably will not work deviates from that standard of competence.
3. Physicians also are obligated to represent standards of scientific knowledge truthfully to the public, claiming neither more nor less than what medicine can actually deliver. Reasonable people will conclude that if a physician offers a treatment, it must have some chance of working. Thus, physicians who employ futile treatments risk becoming quacks or frauds.
4. Physicians are justified in risking harm to patients only when the possible benefit strongly outweighs the risk. If benefit is practically zero, there can be no justification for any risk of harm. Demanding futile treatments, especially those, such as CPR, that can cause pain, forces physicians to become agents of harm, not benefit.

I conclude that physicians should not be forced to provide treatments reliably determined to be futile, as that would force them to violate the dictates of their own professional integrity. We must now ask what practical policies could balance physicians' concerns with maintaining their own integrity against ethical concerns that patients' rights not be trampled in the process.

Toward practical futility policies

We have seen why the concept of futility has proven so complex and perplexing yet carries so much moral weight that it cannot be dismissed. Let us conclude by asking a final set of questions: does the problem get worse when we stop talking in generalities and start talking about real cases with real persons? Or might it be that the abstraction itself has caused some of the problem, so that once we deal with specifics, the view actually becomes clearer?

Recall that in discussing CPR, I suggested two things: first, that when we looked at the relatively abstract question of whether physicians could unilaterally decide DNAR status, the debate was intense and intractable; and second, that when we looked at an issue with undeniably practical implications – whether physicians should unilaterally decide whether and when to stop CPR – most of the debate melted away. That example gives us some hope that the descent from the general to the particular will improve our understanding of futility in practice.

Tomlinson and Czlonka (1995) offer one particularly well-developed approach to a futility policy for a health care institution. A brief summary of the key points of their policy is provided in Table 1.1, but such a synopsis does not really do justice to their insights into how a futility policy actually should work. They understand quite well that in the practical setting, many of the issues that most vex the philosopher or the theoretician recede into the background, and other issues move to center stage.

For instance, it would seem absolutely essential to define futility precisely and consistently before developing a policy on how to deal with it. A good part of the wisdom of Tomlinson and Czlonka's policy lies in refusing to take this approach. To a degree, the response to the demand for a definition is like that of the proverbial baseball umpire, who, on being asked whether the previous pitch was a ball or a strike, replied, "It ain't nothin' till I call it." For practical policy purposes, the question ceases to be "What are the necessary and sufficient conditions for a medical intervention to be said to be futile?" and becomes "How should we resolve disputes over what medical interventions should be deemed futile?" A fair and thoughtful mechanism for dispute resolution turns out to have far more value in the real world than a philosophically elegant definition.

Underlying this aspect of the policy is a deeper insight. Opponents of the concept of futility charge that unilateral futility judgments are an unacceptable abuse of the physician's power over the patient or family. Futility defenders respond by trying to define futility ever more precisely, which in turn leads the opponents to charge that the fancy definitions merely conceal the abuse of power. Tomlinson and Czlonka, by contrast, accept that futility judgments involve the exercise of power by physicians. The question then becomes how to monitor and supervise that use of power and resolve disagreements evenhandedly when abuse is charged.

One way to summarize the wisdom of a practical approach to futility decisions in medicine is to turn to the metaphor of *conversation*. Conversation, in the view of Katz (1984), is useful for better understanding informed consent. What might at first seem a legal fiction unrelated to medicine can be reconceptualized as a vital component of medical practice once physicians

Table 1.1 *Outline of a hospital policy on futile CPR*

1. Definition: *Futile*, provides no meaningful possibility of extended life or other benefit for the patient.
2. Physician (with appropriate specialty consultation) makes preliminary determination that attempted resuscitation would be futile or harmful for a given patient.
3. Attending physician informs competent patient, or surrogate for an incompetent patient, when a preliminary determination of futility has been made. Physician explains reasoning and seeks concurrence with decision not to attempt CPR.
4. If patient or surrogate concurs, physician documents discussion and enters DNAR order.
5. If patient or surrogate does not concur, physician seeks input of ethics committee consultation team to
   a Evaluate correctness of futility determination,
   b Aid with communication and negotiation process.
6. If ethics consultation team supports physician, and patient or family continues to disagree, physicians or hospital try to identify another physician within or outside of facility willing to assume care under conditions specified.
7. If transfer of care cannot be arranged, case goes back to full ethics committee for review and final disposition, in concert with legal counsel if needed.
8. Implementation of policy requires extensive and ongoing staff education around futility issues.

Source: Adapted from Tomlinson and Czlonka 1995.

realize that informed consent is an invitation to have a certain type of conversation with their patients. Katz deliberately used the homely word ''conversation'' instead of a more technical term to demystify what had seemed to many an arcane debate: one need not be a lawyer or an ethicist to comprehend what it means for a doctor to talk with a patient about a treatment decision.

Consider situations in which physicians are talking with patients (or surrogates) about what treatment ought to be used. Such a circumstance requires one of at least three different sorts of conversations. One type of conversation will be by far the most common, but occasionally other considerations will require the conversation to assume one of the other two forms.

The physician's side of the first and by far most common form of conversation goes roughly like this.

The autonomy conversation
''You have a disease, and the treatment options for this disease are the following. Each one (including no treatment) has consequences that might be either good or bad for you. I'd like to describe these consequences to you, along with some idea of how likely or unlikely each one is, so that you can

decide which treatment option would best promote your overriding values. If you want, I can list the options and their consequences in a neutral fashion and leave the decision totally up to you. Or, if you prefer, I can offer advice and suggestions as we go along. The goal of this conversation is to allow you to make an informed choice of a treatment option, taking as active a role in the decision as you wish.''

This could also be dubbed the ''informed consent conversation.'' It assumes that patient autonomy is the operative principle and generally trumps competing principles.

The other two, less frequent conversations are called for when it appears, at least at first glance, that some other moral principle might outweigh respect for patient autonomy. As we have seen, one such competing principle is respect for professional integrity. Another competing principle, increasingly important in an era of scarce resources and fixed budgets, is justice. Issues of justice have arisen for a long time in deciding who gets to be first in line for transplant organs or who gets the last bed when the intensive care unit is full. Today, these issues also arise commonly in managed care settings, when explicit decisions have to be made about whether a patient will receive a very expensive treatment that offers little if any benefit. Since Lo and others are concerned that resource scarcity will be linked inappropriately to futility, it is critical to distinguish these two conversations carefully. They go roughly as follows.

The futility conversation
''You seem to have settled on a decision to request or demand a certain medical intervention. I have a problem with this choice. As best as I can tell, this particular intervention will not succeed in achieving the goals that I presume you want to pursue with regard to your health. So first I have to explore with you the facts about your present situation, as it appears likely that your choice of this intervention is based simply on not knowing these facts. If we find that the discussion of the facts doesn't cause you to change your mind, our conversation will have to take a new direction. Perhaps you can show me that you are trying to pursue a goal different from the one I had assumed; or perhaps you reject my facts and want to get another opinion. In either case, I feel obligated to let you know that what you are asking of me seems to require me to do something that I consider to be bad medical practice. Possibly, our ongoing conversation will show me that I am wrong, but I want you to understand why I am raising this issue and why I feel strongly about the matter – not to be disrespectful of you and your choice but rather to fulfill my professional obligations.''

The justice conversation

"You seem to have settled on a decision to request or demand a certain medical intervention. I have no problem with this choice insofar as it seems to be a rational choice for you and to offer you some prospect of benefit. But the role I play [for instance, as a primary physician working within an HMO plan] has imposed on me certain obligations – not only to you but also to other patients who might need scarce or expensive treatment. According to the rules or standards of this system [such as an HMO's benefit package], you don't seem to me to qualify. I need to explain to you why I think this, and you might then wish to challenge my reasoning. If you and I can't agree, I need to tell you about the mechanisms for appeal that you may use, especially if you think that any form of inappropriate bias has entered into my decision or that I am not adequately informed about all aspects of the treatment that you want. I'm sorry to have to take this position, but I feel forced into it because the duty I owe to you is balanced against the duty that I owe to other patients."

Four points about these conversations are especially important. First, it is important to understand the difference between the futility (integrity) conversation and the justice conversation, as at least some futility advocates seem to think that they are basically the same (Murphy 1994). Treatment that is of small benefit and that is very costly might appropriately be provided to the patient if for some reason it were to become much cheaper, but treatment that violates the physician's professional integrity does so regardless of its cost. If one is principally concerned about justice, it is important to identify which treatments are futile, as it seems totally unjust to withhold a potentially beneficial treatment from one patient while another patient gets a treatment of no benefit whatsoever. It does not follow, however, that if one is principally concerned about professional integrity, one must consider the cost or relative scarcity of the treatment or make any comparative judgments between the degree of entitlement of different patients.

The second point is that the futility conversation is not the autonomy conversation. Some would argue that futility conversations are never necessary because in almost all cases we could accomplish everything we want by using the autonomy conversation, and by phrasing the futility conversation to indicate where it overlaps partially with autonomy (that is, the hope that a clearer explanation of the facts will lead the patient voluntarily to renounce the treatment originally requested). There is something deceptive about trying to characterize the futility conversation as a form of the autonomy conversation, however, because a different moral principle is at stake. In the futility conversation, the physician accurately informs the patient that there is a conflict. If the futility conversation were replaced with an autonomy conversation, the professional integrity issues would be obscured.

Third, putting futility into conversation form may help to defuse some of the fears of the opponents. To some degree, almost all of the objections to the futility concept come down to the fear that it will provide physicians with a license to do things (or to fail to do things) to patients without bothering to talk to the patients about them. (This is why the term ''unilateral'' stirs up so much heat.) If calling an intervention ''futile'' requires that the ethical physician engage in a special sort of conversation with the patient, we seem to have a reasonable safeguard that full and frank discussions will occur. If a futility policy results in conversations of this type within health care institutions whenever physicians feel compelled to refuse treatment on grounds of futility, the policy may offer reasonable protection to the moral values of both physicians and patients.

The fourth point is closely related to the third. The danger in futility determinations is the abuse of physician power. In futility conversations, physicians state clearly what power they propose to exercise, on what authority they feel entitled to exercise it, and what checks and balances ensure that these exercises of power do not constitute abuses. The physicians also remind the patients, as part of the conversation, about the countervailing sources of power they possesses (such as a right to a second medical opinion, ethics committee review, and so on). Under these circumstances, it seems hard to imagine how the power to determine futility could be abused on a regular basis. Of course in some settings, both futility conversations and autonomy conversations might be nonexistent or perfunctory. Up to this point, I have assumed that U.S. health care institutions have learned the autonomy lesson of the last quarter-century and strive to involve patients or surrogates in key decisions about care, including end-of-life issues. Sadly, some data show that this is far from universal (Solomon et al. 1993; SUPPORT Principal Investigators 1995). Inadequate attention to patient autonomy is not a good reason to dismiss the concept of futility, however. Instead, it calls for a more careful distinction of whether autonomy or futility is the basis of the conversation we ought to have. Indeed, better understanding of futility may indirectly spur enhanced respect for autonomy, as the principle of autonomy is both more understandable and more acceptable to physicians once they see its proper limits.

Conclusion

This chapter reviews reasons why the concept of futility has proved so perplexing for medical ethicists. As long as we try to subsume all futility considerations under the principles of autonomy or justice and demand abstract but precise definitions, we are likely to remain muddled. In contrast, once we realize that the ethical principle of professional integrity plays a pivotal role, that futility judgments should start rather than stop conversations among physicians, patients, and families, and that most of the difficult problems are matters of practical policy, we may find ourselves on firm ground.

References

Brody, H. 1994. The physician's role in determining futility. *Journal of the American Geriatrics Society* 42:875–8.

Katz, J. 1984. *The Silent World of Doctor and Patient.* New York: Free Press.

Lo, B. 1995. Futile interventions. In *Resolving Ethical Dilemmas: A Guide for Clinicians*, pp. 73–81. Baltimore: Williams & Wilkins.

Miller, F.G., and Brody, H. 1995. Professional integrity and physician-assisted death. *Hastings Center Report* 25(May–June):8–17.

Moss, A.H. 1989. Informing the patient about cardiopulmonary resuscitation: when the risks outweigh the benefits. *Journal of General Internal Medicine* 4:349–55.

Murphy, D.J. 1994. Can we set futile care policies? Institutional and systemic challenges. *Journal of the American Geriatrics Society* 42:890–3.

Pellegrino, E.D., and Thomasma, D.C. 1981. *A Philosophical Basis of Medical Practice.* New York: Oxford University Press.

Schneiderman, L.J., and Jecker, N.S. 1995. *Wrong Medicine: Doctors, Patients, and Futile Treatment.* Baltimore: Johns Hopkins University Press.

Schneiderman, L.J., Jecker, N.S., and Jonsen, A.R. 1990. Medical futility: its meaning and ethical implications. *Annals of Internal Medicine* 112:949–54.

Solomon, M.Z., O'Donnell, L., Jennings, B., et al. 1993. Decisions near the end of life: professional views on life-sustaining treatment. *American Journal of Public Health* 83:14–23.

SUPPORT Principal Investigators. 1995. A controlled trial to improve care for seriously ill hospital patients. The Study to Understand Prognoses and Preferences for Outcomes and Risks of Treatment (SUPPORT). *Journal of the American Medical Association* 274:1591–8.

Tomlinson, T., and Czlonka, D. 1995. Futility and hospital policy. *Hastings Center Report* 25(May–June):28–35.

Veatch, R.M. 1973. Generalization of expertise. *Hastings Center Studies* 1(Mar–Apr):29–40.

Waisel, D.B., and Truog, R.D. 1995. The cardiopulmonary-resuscitation-not-indicated order. *Annals of Internal Medicine* 122:304–8.

2

Death with dignity?

PATRICIA BROPHY, R.N.

I was told by two physicians in 1985 that there was no such thing as death with dignity. They were the then president of the Massachusetts Citizens for Life, Dr. Joseph Stanton, and the physician-in-chief of the New England Sinai Hospital, Dr. Richard Field. I vehemently disagreed with them. The following story explains my position.

Paul Brophy was the youngest of nine children in an Irish Catholic family. His mother, with her famous Irish wit, described her family as three and a half dozen children. You may ask "How can that be?" Well, there were three girls and a half dozen boys.

I knew Paul since we were children. We lived exactly a mile apart. We attended the same church and Sunday School. We became good friends in high school, began dating, eventually married, and had a large, Irish Catholic family of our own. Paul was a healthy, hearty person who loved life, family, and work. In his spare time, he especially enjoyed hunting, fishing, camping, and gardening, in that order. He had been a firefighter and emergency medical technician (EMT) with the fire department in Easton, Massachusetts. He was an active member of the Easton Permanent Firefighters Association, president of the Association for two terms, and an integral part of its negotiating team. When it came to negotiating the fire department contract with the town, he possessed a fierce and competitive spirit.

We had been married nearly 25 years and Paul was 45 years old when tragedy struck. Paul came to bed the night of March 22, 1983, grabbed his head and said, "I have a splitting headache," and passed out. Our world ended in the twinkling of an eye.

I could not arouse him. The EMTs with whom Paul worked responded to my emergency call. Paul regained consciousness when being moved but was disoriented to time, place, and occurring events. He was transported to the emergency room at Goddard Hospital, where it was determined that he had

15

suffered a ruptured brain aneurysm. After transfer to the neurologic intensive care unit (ICU) of the New England Medical Center in Boston, he was kept in a stimulation-deprived environment for 10 days while the blood around his brain dissipated and the brain swelling subsided. This was to ensure the best conditions for operating and clipping the aneurysm.

As I reflect, I realize that those 10 days were a gift from God. Throughout the turmoil of illness, not knowing what was happening, I was somehow deeply touched by just being there, sitting by his bed, holding his hand, and encouraging him. This cemented the already strong bond between us. Little did I realize that this was one of the many ways in which the Lord was strengthening me for the three and a half years of anguish that lay ahead.

A craniotomy was performed on April 6, 1983. The surgery was successful, but vasospasms after the surgery caused a massive stroke, and Paul never regained consciousness. For the next three and a half years, he remained in a coma that evolved into a persistent vegetative state.

Following three months of acute care, Paul was transferred to New England Sinai Hospital, a chronic care facility, just 10 miles from our home. I chose this facility because of its location. I could go each day to help Paul in his rehabilitation. I could be involved in his care until I could bring him home. So I thought – and hoped.

When Paul arrived at Sinai, he was being nourished via a nasogastric tube. He also had a tracheostomy with oxygen mist to facilitate breathing. As time passed, Sinai asked my permission to insert a gastrostomy tube because the nasogastric tube was causing pneumonia and other respiratory problems. The doctor also stressed the possibility of permanent damage to the larynx from the nasogastric tube. I gave my permission for insertion of the gastrostomy tube, not having an inkling of what I was about to face.

Days passed; weeks turned into months. There were many hugs and tears, but more than anything else, still hope – hope that today would be the day Paul would wake up. People stopped asking, stopped visiting; it was as though he was gone. Well, he was, yet he lingered. His hands curled in, and his arms grew stiff. His legs that once were strong from running were now like twigs. They were curling up and contracting more each day. He wore sneakers to prevent footdrop. It was so sad, so very painful to watch this man who, a few months ago, had been vital, happy, and healthy.

He was such a strong person, with a strong heart, and he lingered on. For many frustrating months, I stood at the foot of his bed, watching him wither, wondering why. Why did this happen to Paul? Why did this happen to us – we are good people, faithful to each other and to our God. Why did the vasospasms occur after a fairly successful operation? Why does he not respond – he was such a healthy person before the aneurysm burst. Why are my prayers not being answered? I discovered later that my prayers were being answered. They just were not answered in the way I had hoped.

Late at night, alone with my thoughts, I would search for answers that would not come. Then I stopped asking why; instead, I began to scream it. It did not make any sense. The hurt, the anger, and the pain would not go away.

Meanwhile, more grandchildren were born into the family. Other family members died. Time marched on for everyone but Paul. People no longer asked about him, or if they did, it was in the past tense. I wanted to take them by the shoulders and shake them. He is not dead! But he was no longer alive, either.

Nearly a year and a half into Paul's illness, the hospital inititated an eight-week program for families of head-injured patients. It was given by a retired psychologist, Dr. Yager, who had recently lost his wife to cancer. In the course of the program, he said he had not allowed the insertion of a feeding tube into his wife. He also very bluntly said, ''Don't you realize your loved ones are going to die? They will never recover.'' This statement hit me like a ton of bricks. I had prayed and prayed for a miracle to happen. But the Lord did not change the situation I was in; He used the situation to change me!

The most unselfish act of love is the ability to let go of someone you love. Paul was a father, son, brother, husband, and friend to so many. We all loved him in our own very special way. He, in turn, enriched all our lives with his specialness – his strength and guidance, his ability to make tough decisions and stick to them. It might have been easier for me to allow things to continue as they were. Many families do. Yet the conflict inside me kept urging, prodding. ''This isn't right.'' Days and months spread into years of grief that did not end.

New England Sinai Hospital never had what I would call a friendly atmosphere, even before I made my decision to let Paul die. The nurses and attendants were so constantly busy that it was impossible for them to spend quality time with families. I never had much contact with social workers or other hospital personnel and found the most comfort from meeting and talking with other families informally and attending the Tuesday afternoon Catholic Mass with Paul. After the first three weeks of Paul's internment, all rehabilitation programs were stopped, and he was on chronic maintenance care. The nursing care Paul received at Sinai was, for the most part, good. However, I believe this was so because I was so constantly there and never silent about care when it was lacking.

I began asking myself questions. What is the difference between being terminally ill and irreversibly ill – in this case, in a persistent vegetative state? A terminally ill person, in 1984, could legally, morally, and ethically have all treatment stopped or not started, whereas a person in a persistent vegetative state had to be nourished with artificial, chemical nutrition and hydration. What moral obligation did Paul have to live in this state? Why must his death be prolonged? When treatment received is not bringing about recovery, why can it not be stopped? Why is it more moral not to start a treatment than to stop ineffective therapy?

I reflected on Paul's life values. After being married to him for 25 years and knowing him since childhood, I thought I knew my husband well – his values, his lifestyle, the things he valued most in life, his strengths, and, God knows, his faults. I gradually realized that his condition was contrary to his beliefs and values. Many times during his life, he had referred to similar situations, starting with the well-known Karen Ann Quinlan case of the seventies. Here he was, in exactly the same condition. I was completely convinced that Paul would never, never want to live like this.

I finally came to the conclusion that I had three choices: do nothing, walk away and forget that Paul existed, or step out in faith and do what I knew Paul would expect me to do as his wife – stop the tube feedings and allow him to die. Emotionally, all of Paul's family and friends were dying, a piece at a time. I approached my pastor and asked his guidance. He gave me not only guidance, but his blessing and support for a decision that I could be at peace with. This decision came through much counseling and prayer. One of the scripture verses that served as a guideline was *Micah*, Ch. 6, V. 8. ''This is what Yahweh expects of you, only this – to love tenderly, act justly, and walk humbly with your God.''

The final decision came after we brought Paul home for Christmas in 1984. We thought that if anything would stimulate him, it would be his own home environment. This was our last shot. Our sons went to the hospital and brought home his adapted wheelchair. The EMTs with whom he had worked transported him in their ambulance. We were so hopeful. His family and friends came and went all day. The grandchildren were running around, climbing onto and bumping into his wheelchair. It turned out to be a living wake; Paul did not respond at all. When the firefighters came and took him back to the hospital, my kids and I stood on the front porch, in zero degree weather, and sobbed. We knew now that he would never return. Hope had lingered its longest hour. The frustration had turned the ''whys'' into ''whats.'' What can I do to change the situation? It was up to me to do what I could for him now.

I tried to pick up the pieces of my life, but the whole situation clouded my mind. I realized with startling clarity that I was not going away from the problem. So I stiffened my backbone and prepared to fight. In my heart I knew what he wanted, and I knew I was right.

I tried to picture him as he had been, happy and healthy. My favorite memories swirled around, but I could not see his face clearly any more, except in pictures. A panic set in; he's going away. He lies alone at night, too, but unaware. I will not fail him. I can hold onto the strength I shared in his love, and hope and pray that someday he will give me a hug. A hug for believing, for not leaving him alone in the past like so many have urged me to do. A hug for not forcing him to live in a life with no hope.

I found myself sharing funny memories with him. I shared them with other family members and close friends, and I could finally laugh at some without rushing from the room to catch my breath. Dreams of panic washed through me at night. I ran from the pain, the anger, the hurt. I had come to realize I could only run so far. The doctors at Sinai wished that I would run away forever and forget, move on, whatever, as long as I did not cause them any discomfort or disrupt their sterile world. But I could not run any more.

I finally opened my heart to a church friend. He, in turn, helped me to contact Father John Paris, who introduced me to attorney Frank Reardon and Dr. Ronald Cranford. These three people became the backbone of my case. I now realize that when I surrendered an impossible situation to the Lord, he began to open doors.

The decision was made to help Paul – to let him die. His life had been over for quite some time now. It was January 1985, and Paul's condition had not changed in almost two years. I searched my soul for the millionth time, looked for guidance from elders and support from family, friends, and church community. Confusion was constant, as many people just did not understand. My five children, Paul's entire family of seven brothers and sisters, and his 90-year-old mother gave me their undivided support. I asked Paul's doctor to stop tube feedings. He refused. Attorney Reardon contacted Dr. Field and asked for a meeting, which he flatly refused, stating there was nothing to talk about. He refused to communicate with us in any way. So, on February 6, 1985, we petitioned the Norfolk County Probate Court for declaratory relief to stop tube feedings. The doctor was furious that I had gone to court, and from that day forward, we received a cold shoulder from all but a few of the hospital staff.

In early May, we came before Judge Kopelman for a hearing. He was not satisfied with the setup, which included an attorney for the hospital, an attorney for me, and a guardian ad litem to research the facts of the case. The judge said that Paul also had a right to counsel, and an attorney was ap-

pointed. This pitted me against my husband. Wait! There is something wrong
with this picture! I find myself in a triangle; everybody's fighting over him:
the hospital, the court-appointed attorney who does not even know him, and
me. And Paul lies there, unaware, lingering. I have lost him once before; I
know how much it hurts. Why do they not see that I am doing this for Paul?
They try to figure out what I have to gain, while I try to figure out how I
am going to survive this experience. The ball is in my court, however, and
I am taking my best shot. The ball has bounced into a court of law.

There are two places I can think of where people do not like to be – in a
hospital and in a courtroom; and we were in both places at once. The emotional strain was wearing us out. In the courtroom, we needed to clarify four
things: diagnosis, prognosis, substituted judgment (what would Paul want),
and family's wishes. The opposition, backed by the Massachusetts Citizens
for Life and other national right to life groups, needed to prove three of the
state's four interests: preservation of life, prevention of suicide, and preservation of the integrity of the medical profession.

We were persecuted by pro-life-backed testimony in the courtroom and in
the media. They called us abusive, cruel, inhumane, and no better than Nazi
murderers. They painted a picture of starvation: lips cracked, eyes sunken in
the sockets, tongue swollen and stuck to the mouth. This nearly destroyed
me. Pro-life forces did not seem to realize that I had opted for life all the
way until we came to the end of the road. When the Lord showed me there
was no life and no hope of recovery, I knew that I had to surrender Paul to
his Creator. I had to stop pumping him full of artificial, chemical nutrition.
I tried and tried to explain this. More than anything else in the world, I
wanted him back – we all did – but it had been two years!

Prior to Paul's illness, we had discussed living wills. There was no legislation in place in Massachusetts at the time, but we had decided that when
it became legal, we would each execute one. Until then, we knew what we
each wanted, so there would be no problem. This was a grave mistake on
our part. It was emphasized in the courtroom that something in writing might
have been taken into consideration. Nevertheless, as the Bible states in *Ro-
mans* Ch. 8, V. 28, ''We know that, in everything, God works for good with
those who love Him, who are called according to His purpose.''

One distressing thing in the courtroom was the fact that, after the family
finished testifying, Paul Brophy was no longer considered. He was lost in a
debate of two factions: the right to life and the right to die. At this point, I
felt like a scapegoat, a pawn in a battle of ideologies.

Five months later, the lower court's ruling was handed down (*Brophy v.
New England Sinai Hospital, Inc.* 1985). The court agreed with the substi-

tuted judgment issue. Judge Kopelman ruled that Paul would not want to live in this condition, but the quality of treatment was more important than the quality of life. We were disappointed but not surprised. My attorney had prepared us for the denial. The important issue was the substituted judgment issue, and the judge had agreed to that. We, as a family, were more determined than ever to go on, and we filed an appeal.

The Supreme Judicial Court of Massachusetts heard oral arguments in March 1986. Its ruling came out in September (*Brophy v. New England Sinai Hospital, Inc.* 1986). We had now been in the court system for a year and a half, and Paul had been in a persistent vegetative state for three and a half years. Try to imagine yourself waking up every day for one and a half years, wondering, is this the day? In the meantime, trying to go on with life, working, visiting Paul, feeling, at times, a failure.

The lower court's decision was turned over by a 4–3 vote. Yes, we could discontinue feedings, but the hospital would not be forced to do so if it was against its policy. However, they were instructed to help us find a willing facility and transfer Paul there. As the hospital had not been cooperative in the past, neither were they now. This was a most horrendous experience. An irreversible comatose husband whom I loved dearly, one and a half years in courts, and a hospital that fought us every step of the way.

Paul's physician, Dr. Konz, was interviewed by a medical magazine. He said that most families of head-injured patients fade away after a while, but Mrs. Brophy had become part of the furniture. Somehow, he did not realize or had not been taught that the family is the extension of the patient.

While we were making arrangements to transfer Paul to Emerson Hospital in Concord, Paul's court-appointed attorney appealed the case to the U.S. Supreme Court in Washington, DC. It was refused.

Paul was transferred to Emerson Hospital on October 15, 1986. I had no idea what to expect after what I had been through at Sinai, but the staff actually talked to me as if I were a normal person. I was treated with compassion, emotional support, and, most of all, with respect for the agonizing decision that I had made. Going from Sinai to Emerson was like going to another planet. Everything that Sinai did wrong, Emerson did right. A cot was brought into Paul's room where I was allowed to stay 24 hours a day. I spent days watching the Red Sox playoffs on TV. The priests from my parish came in to support us. Friends sent cards. My five children were awesome. My brother and his wife even flew in from Texas to be near. The head nurse on Paul's team was hospice-trained. She realized the importance of family involvement. I was allowed to take part in both medical decision making and hands-on nursing care during the dying process.

This final phase of Paul's life was the most difficult yet the most rewarding eight days of my life. Paul died a peaceful death on October 23, 1986. I emphasize peaceful. It was not a death of starvation as painted in the courtroom. During those last eight days, Paul's physical condition deteriorated, and he eventually contracted pneumonia, dying peacefully. His physical appearance actually became more like his former self. He lost the facial bloating that had resulted from the forced feedings. It was almost as if time was reversing itself. It was now Paul in the bed, dying naturally, and not some artificial image of the Paul who Sinai wanted to believe was there, yet was not. The grandchildren came and played on his bed. They were not afraid of him. They kissed him goodbye because he was going to heaven. He died peacefully, surrounded by his family, loving and committed to the end.

What are some of the things I have learned from this experience? First, we need to realize that people are physical, emotional, psychologic, and spiritual beings. Every aspect of our complex nature needs nurturing. Perhaps the operative definitions of death are not sufficient in today's society. When did Paul stop being a person? Had he stopped being a person? He certainly stopped being Paul. Why was he not considered terminally ill when there was no hope of recovery? I remember sitting beside his bed asking, ''Where are you, Paul? Are you in or out of your body? Are you in a tunnel between life and death? Do you have the door to eternity open, and we are holding you back? Or are you in complete darkness, like a long sleep, waiting to be let go to your eternal destination?''

As a result of this experience, my philosophy on the meaning of death emerged. It is different and probably a bit more liberal than some. I believe that a quality of life must be factored into the whole picture of life on earth. I lean toward Robert Veatch, who says that ''Death means a complete change in the status of a living entity characterized by the irreversible loss of those characteristics that are essentially significant to it'' (Veatch, 1976:25). However, with the advent of technology, the body can be nourished for an unpredictable number of years while the cortex of the brain does not work. This is an unacceptable definition of life to me.

Death is not a failure. It is the fulfillment of life. It is an opening to a changed life. If I lose my ability to think, to respond to my environment inside or outside of my body, then I am not living. Body, mind, and spirit must be integrated. When the cerebral cortex dies, there will never again be integration of mind and body. I am not sure where the spirit fits into the picture. Perhaps, at this point it is straining to be freed.

Death is being medicalized and legalized in our society. The movement toward legalizing physician-assisted suicide has become a definite threat.

Contrary to popular belief, much can be done for the dying. Physicians, patients, and families can continue to learn how and when to withhold or withdraw technical interventions that are burdensome and degrading to the sanctity of life. Stopping ineffective therapy and allowing death to occur naturally seems compatible with respect for life.

The Washington Catholic Bishops adopted arguments against euthanasia, adding the admonition of Father Richard McCormack that those who insist that life support systems must be used at all times, even though the patient will not benefit, could well be unwittingly contributing to public acceptance of active euthanasia. People cringe at the thought of dying a prolonged death. They are aware of the Karen Ann Quinlans, the Paul Brophys, and the Nancy Cruzans of this world, who lingered on hopelessly year after year.

Although much legislation is in place today to help people avoid the predicament of *Brophy*, society has a long way to go to provide a consensus of acceptable behavior about right-to-life/right-to-die issues.

I hope that my family's experience has helped society to move toward resolution of the ongoing struggle of families caught in the turmoil of life and death issues.

Reference

Veatch, R.M. 1976. *Death, Dying and the Biological Revolution.* New Haven and London: Yale University Press.

Cases

Brophy v. New England Sinai Hospital, Inc., No. 85E0009-G1 (Mass. Probate and Family Court, Oct. 21, 1985) (Kopelman, J.)
Brophy v. New England Sinai Hospital, Inc., 398 Mass. 417, 497 N.E. 2d 626 (1986).

3

Physicians and medical futility: experience in the critical care setting

HARRY S. RAFKIN, M.D., AND
THOMAS RAINEY, M.D.

Intensive care units were created to facilitate and enhance the delivery of care to the most extremely ill patients. Underlying this concept was the assumption that grouping critically ill patients in one area staffed by physicians and nurses trained in the care of such patients would improve the delivery of care. This approach has been effective. Despite the high level of illness seen in the intensive care unit (ICU), hospital mortality rates for ICU patients range from 15% to 20%.

Paradoxically, the advances that have allowed a high survival rate have also created an increase in the number of individuals who survive in a state of chronic persistent illness. Many of these patients proceed to a slow death at the expense of both human suffering and dollars spent. As a consequence, the process of dying has been scrutinized as closely as other more traditional aspects of health care delivery. How we die in the ICU has become an issue.

The public has become more sophisticated about the strengths and weaknesses of critical care and is asking more frequently that physicians not administer care that fails to confer benefit to the patient. Similarly, some physicians have become more sophisticated about the limitations of medical care and about the suffering that can result from invasive, yet unfruitful, therapy and are now less willing to administer care that they consider of no benefit, even in the rare circumstances when they are asked to do so.

Thus, the public is less willing to accept futile care, and physicians are less willing to deliver it. Despite this apparent concordance, the issue of futile care remains problematic. At the moment of initial intervention, we are unable to predict which patients will recover and which will not. Furthermore, care given at the outset to those who do not ultimately survive is not futile in that everyone emotionally involved needs to feel that everything worthwhile has been done. Thus, futile care remains difficult to define and to identify at an early stage of the disease process.

At later stages of critical illness, the effectiveness of care may become clearer. The goals of therapy may change, and therapy can be modified to meet these goals. Therefore, physicians and patients must develop a process through which care can be continually reassessed as the disease process evolves. The decision to withdraw or withhold therapy in critically ill patients is complex, requiring not only an in-depth understanding of the patient's medical condition but also an intimate understanding of the patient's desires and those of the family. The intensive care specialist must be able to process this information to orchestrate and deliver expert care not only when patients survive but also when death becomes inevitable.

It must be kept in mind that physicians and patients will bring to the process a spectrum of personal and religious values. Although the corpus of thought in medical ethics in the United States considers withdrawing and withholding care as ethically similar, not all individuals or groups agree. For example, Orthodox Jews hold that these two processes are not equivalent ethically, and consequently, they approach end-of-life decisions differently. In all circumstances, the physician must be able to assess the medical prognosis accurately and realistically and allow the patient or health care proxy to make appropriate decisions consistent with his or her religious or personal convictions. If the physician does not agree with the ethical values of the patient and wishes to withdraw from the case, the physician should find another who will guide the patient in end-of-life decisions.

We review several entities responsible for a major proportion of deaths in the ICU and discuss accepted mechanisms for withdrawing or withholding life support when medical therapy is considered futile.

Outcome in selected clinical entities

Relation of age to outcome

Rockwood et al. (1993) carried out a year-long prospective analysis of 1,040 patients in intensive care. Differences in outcome were associated with severity of illness, length of stay, prior ICU admission, and respiratory failure, but not with age. Follow-up interviews with one-year survivors revealed that activities of daily living were the same for the elderly patients and the younger subgroup. Self-perception of the level of health status did not differ between the two groups. However, only 7% of the elderly patients with a functional limitation in these activities were unhappy, whereas 15% of the younger patients were unhappy and felt that the ICU admission had not been worthwhile.

Thus, age should not be used as a criterion for determining the potential benefit of critical care. Moreover, elderly patients appear psychologically more tolerant of functional impairments that may accrue as a consequence of their illness and view the ICU experience as worthwhile.

Cardiac arrest in the elderly

Cardiac resuscitation is an area of significant research in critical care medicine, and recommendations are revised periodically. The procedure requires insertion of a tube for breathing, chest compression, and, frequently, insertion of large-bore venous catheters for intravascular access. Although the patient is unconscious during the process and cannot experience pain, the procedure carries with it a great degree of physical invasiveness and violation of physical dignity.

A retrospective analysis of 114 patients who received cardiopulmonary resuscitation (CPR) in an ICU showed that 70% of patients were successfully resuscitated, but only 11% survived to discharge from the hospital (Peterson et al. 1991). Hypotension in the prearrest period, sepsis, severe disease, and long duration of CPR correlated with a poor outcome. Those who were discharged to home had a median survival of 42 months.

In light of the low rate of survival in such patients, it would be useful to identify prospectively which patients have a higher probability of survival when CPR is conducted. Landry, Parker, and Phillips (1992) addressed this question in a retrospective study of 114 ICU patients and hypothesized that severe chronic disease would influence outcome from CPR. Malignancy was noted in 29% of these patients, vascular disease in 20%, chronic liver disease in 7%, end stage liver disease in 5%, chronic obstructive pulmonary disease in 5%, and other conditions in 34%. Although nearly half the patients were initially resuscitated, only six survived to discharge. Of these six, only two were alive at one year, and both had severe disabilities. Not one of the patients with malignancy or sepsis survived the initial CPR.

A prospective study of 477 patients in a Dutch ICU showed that although 47% survived CPR, only 3% survived to discharge (Miranda 1994). Survivors showed some dysfunction in psychosocial interactions, as well as progressive deterioration of mental function, particularly with regard to awareness of the environment. Alertness, appetite, and the capacity for resuming work were all diminished compared to the patient's pre-CPR status.

In summary, ICU patients who experience cardiac arrest have a generally poor survival rate. Survival is influenced by the general condition of the patient before the cardiac arrest, and quality of life in survivors frequently is diminished.

Sepsis and multisystem organ failure

Sepsis, or invasion of the blood by microorganisms, can lead to hypotension, referred to as "septic shock." Sepsis can also produce multisystem organ failure, a syndrome characterized by dysfunction of two or more organs. Both these entities have high mortality rates. Thus, among 700 patients with sepsis, the crude mortality rate was 18.8%. The death rate caused by sepsis without coexisting medical problems was 6.9%, but the rate was 52.2% in the presence of septic shock (Haug et al. 1994).

Many patients with sepsis may survive initially but succumb shortly after discharge. Sasse et al. (1995) prospectively analyzed 153 patients with sepsis. The hospital mortality rate was 51%, but the mortality rates among those discharged were 40.5%, 64.7%, and 71.9%. at one month, six months, and one year, respectively. These data suggest that survivors of sepsis have a compromised level of health. Perl et al. (1995) reviewed quality of life issues in 100 patients with sepsis and reported that immediate survivors reported more physical dysfunction at home and in the workplace than among survivors of other serious illnesses.

Multisystem organ failure has a high mortality rate, which correlates with the number of nonfunctional organ systems. Failure of one organ, two organs, and three organs resulted in mortality rates of 40%, 60%, and 98%, respectively (Knaus et al. 1985). Tran et al. (1990) confirmed this relationship.

In summary, the mortality rate for sepsis is close to 20% despite medical advances, and the mortality rate for failure of three organs approaches 100%.

Cancer patients in the ICU

The survival of cancer patients in the ICU has been scrutinized in relation to the high cost of care for these patients. Schapira et al. (1993) evaluated 83 patients with solid tumors and 64 patients with hematologic cancer. Mortality rates in the ICU were 68% and 59% for solid and hematologic cancer, respectively. Patients requiring mechanical ventilation had a mortality rate in the range of 70% for both types of tumors. The cost per year of life gained was $82,854 for patients with solid tumors and $189,339 for those with hematologic tumors.

Because of the cost and the relatively low survival in ICU patients with cancer, the appropriateness of CPR is often questioned. For example, although CPR was successful in 19 of 49 cancer patients, only 5 were discharged from the hospital. CPR was successful in all 8 patients in whom cardiac arrest was the consequence of cardiovascular toxicity, even in the presence of metastatic cancer, but CPR was successful in only 25% of cases when cardiac arrest was a complication of other specific problems, such as septic shock or respiratory failure.

Human immunodeficiency virus (HIV) infection and Pneumocystis carinii *pneumonia (PCP)*

Outcome from HIV-related PCP in ICU patients has been analyzed closely because of the heavy treatment burden placed on these patients. Wachter et al. (1995) analyzed outcome data in 113 patients in three eras: 1981–5, 1986–8, and 1989–91. Survival was 14%, 39%, and 24%, respectively. The average length of hospital stay was 9.5 days, and no difference was noted across the three eras. The increased mortality in 1989–91 caused the cost per year of life saved to escalate from $94,528 in 1986–8 to $215,233. These data suggest that mortality from PCP may be increasing in HIV patients as cost effectiveness of therapy is decreasing. The evolution of this situation will require continued monitoring.

Objective data and forgoing life support

It is apparent that medical therapy in the ICU is often unable to alleviate the underlying disease. Under these circumstances, the needs of the patient change, and many patients and their families request that care be withheld or withdrawn.

Forgoing life support requires that the patient and physician understand the complexities of the situation to the best of their abilities and that they communicate their respective goals. From the physician's perspective, predicting the mortality risk with a reasonable degree of accuracy requires a high degree of familiarity with the medical literature. Although several systems for scoring the severity of disease can be applied objectively to predict mortality for large groups of patients (Knaus et al. 1985; Lemeshow et al. 1993), their applicability to individual risk prediction is highly controversial. Although the mortality rates are high in all of the entities reviewed, they are often considerably less than 100%. Thus, any critically ill patient, given the benefits of invasive and skilled intensive care medicine and the right combination of circumstances, can survive despite the odds. One should, therefore, not be impulsive in proclaiming a given situation irreversible.

The physician must view each patient individually and present a realistic assessment. In attempting to separate potential survivors from nonsurvivors, it is crucial to bear in mind that comorbidity contributes a great deal to the overall prognosis. Patients show marked resilience when their status before the current illness was relatively sound, as survival data in cardiac arrest, sepsis, and oncology patients suggest. Death is more likely when the patient has preexisting medical problems.

Arriving at the conclusion that death is imminent requires a process involving the patient, family, and physician. Daily evaluation of the clinical situation is necessary over a period of days or weeks. Ultimately, a Rubicon is crossed, and the physician considers death to be inescapable. At this time, the nature of care recommended by the physician should change. In no way does care cease; rather priority is given to issues of comfort, time with loved ones, and avoidance of painful procedures, invasive monitoring, and unnecessary testing.

Once it has become clear that further heroic therapy serves only to prolong dying, American jurisprudence and medical ethics deem it admissible to withhold or withdraw therapy aside from that addressing the patient's comfort. The decision to withdraw or withhold specific therapies should be based on discussions, often quite intricate, with the patient, family, or health care proxy where appropriate. During these discussions, the physician relates the professional opinion that the medical condition is irreversible, and the patient, family, or proxy, speaking on behalf of the patient, expresses its wish that therapy be withheld or withdrawn. Under routine circumstances, legal counsel is not required to formalize this process. If there are unclear circumstances, an ethics consultation may be obtained to clarify issues. The form for forgoing life support employed at St. Francis Medical Center is shown in Table 3.1. Essentially any type of therapy that is used in the ICU can be addressed by this form.

Patients not only can request that therapy be withdrawn or withheld but also can request that it be initiated. Thus, a policy for forgoing life support acts as an important vehicle for discussion between the patient or health care proxy and the physician. Because of the severity of illness now commonly seen in the ICU and the relatively high risk of death, it is essential that the patient and physician communicate at an early stage and throughout the evolution of the disease about the patient's wishes and the physician's prognosis.

Table 3.1. *Form used at St. Francis Hospital, Pittsburgh, PA, for forgoing life support*

PATIENT NAME _____ DATE _____
PATIENT'S DIAGNOSIS _____
The following are orders established for the medical care of this patient by Dr. _____
after consultation and in accordance with the wishes of the patient and/or surrogate ____

	YES	NO	NOT APPLICABLE
Mask to Mouth Resuscitation without Intubation	___	___	_____
External Chest Compression	___	___	_____
Electrical Ventricular Defibrillation	___	___	_____
Chemical Ventricular Defibrillation	___	___	_____
Intubation without Mechanical Ventilation	___	___	_____
Intubation with Mechanical Ventilation	___	___	_____

IF ANY OF THE ABOVE SIX (6) ARE CHECKED (X) YES, A CARDIAC ARREST MUST BE CALLED.

	YES	NO	NOT APPLICABLE
Inotropic and Vasoactive Support	___	___	_____
Electrical Cardioversion for Atrial Tachyarrhythmia	___	___	_____
Transfer to ICU	___	___	_____
Dialysis	___	___	_____
Transfusion	___	___	_____
IV Support	___	___	_____
IV Hyperalimentation	___	___	_____
Enteral Nutrition	___	___	_____
Antibiotics	___	___	_____
Chemotherapy	___	___	_____
Radiation Therapy	___	___	_____
Radiologic Studies	___	___	_____
Laboratory Studies	___	___	_____

Informed Consent was obtained from (name or names) _____

Comments: _____

_____   _____
                                       ATTENDING PHYSICIAN'S SIGNATURE

This order should ordinarily be reviewed on a weekly basis and signed by M.D. However, it will remain in effect unless superseded by a subsequent order. If the patient is discharged and readmitted, these orders must be rewritten. However, direct transfers among divisions (General, Psychiatry and Rehabilitation) do not require that the orders be rewritten. They must still be reviewed.
Weekly review dates and physician's signature:

Date _____ _____ M.D.   Date _____ _____ M.D.
Date _____ _____ M.D.   Date _____ _____ M.D.

From the patient's perspective, a basic appreciation of CPR and its limitations facilitates effective discussion with the medical team. Not all patients and families are aware of the poor survival rates of CPR or of its invasiveness. Murphy et al. (1994) evaluated patients' preferences for CPR by interviewing 287 patients with a mean age of 77 in an ambulatory practice. Initially, 41% agreed to accept CPR if it were necessary, but after learning the estimated probability of survival, only 22% chose to have CPR in the event of a cardiac arrest. The percentage choosing CPR was much lower in patients over 86 years of age and those with a chronic illness.

Contemporary procedures for forgoing life support differ significantly from the do not resuscitate (DNR) orders that are written on medical charts by physicians. DNR orders essentially address only the situation in which cardiac arrest occurred. They do not necessarily facilitate communication between patient and physician at an early stage in the disease or permit the patient to make sound medical judgments throughout the course of the disease. With the emphasis on resuscitation, inadequate emphasis was placed on the global disease process. In reality, supportive care in a modern ICU can maintain a critically ill patient in a state of limbo for weeks. Cardiac arrest may not occur, but a state of irreversible critical illness may persist nevertheless. Although individuals may approach this situation differently depending on religious or personal persuasion, the medical community must recognize that withdrawal of therapy is not of necessity illegal or unethical according to the corpus of ethical thought accepted in the United States at present. A recent study by Asch, Hansen-Flaschen, and Lanken (1995) suggested that there is significant misunderstanding about this point.

With a true policy for forgoing life support, therapy at the end of life can be tailored to meet all appropriate needs of the patient, including attention to pain medication, sedation, and specialized nursing care. Thus, we view forgoing life support as a process that engages the patient or health care proxy and the physician in a constructive informative dialogue and allows appropriate decisions concerning treatment options to be made at each stage of the disease.

All states have laws governing forgoing life support (advance directives), and the federal Patient Self-Determination Act requires health care facilities that receive federal support to tell their patients about their right to execute such directives (Yamani et al. 1995). All such facilities, including nursing homes and rehabilitation centers, are required to have a policy for forgoing life support if they wish to be accredited by the Joint Commission on Accreditation of Healthcare Organizations (JCAHO). The JCAHO is a private, not-for-profit, voluntary accrediting agency that is used by most health care facilities. The JCAHO requires that a policy for forgoing life support describe the following: the procedure for reaching a decision about a DNR order, the mechanisms in place for resolving conflicts in decision making, and the role of physicians, nursing staff, other staff, and family members in reaching a DNR order. The policy must include provisions that ensure that the rights of patients are respected. It should be in writing and available to patients and their families on request.

Although policies differ among hospitals, in general any type of order for forgoing life support must be discussed with the patient who is capable of making medical decisions. A problem arises when the ICU patient lacks this capacity. This situation occurs relatively frequently and may be a direct consequence of the disease process or secondary to sedation administered in the ICU. A patient lacking this capacity still has the right to self-determination about health care matters, which can be expressed through an advance directive (living will or appointment of a proxy by executing a medical power of attorney). In about half the states, in the absence of an advance directive, family members or other surrogates are legally empowered to make health care decisions for the patient.

A recent study (SUPPORT Principal Investigators 1995) found serious deficiencies in the willingness of many physicians to talk to seriously ill patients and their families about wishes for treatment at the end of life. This was a two-phase prospective study aimed at improving end-of-life decision making. Phase 1 consisted of a two-year prospective observational study of 4,301 patients, documenting the degree of patient–physician communication, the frequency of aggressive treatment at the end of life, and the characteristics of hospital death. Phase 2 consisted of a two-year controlled trial of 4,810 patients and their physicians randomized to an intervention group or a control group. Physicians in the intervention group received daily estimates of six-month survival, outcomes of CPR, and the estimated functional disability at six months. During phase 1, serious deficiencies were found among physicians in their willingness to talk to patients and their families. The intervention protocol of phase 2 failed to improve communication or patient care. It is thus important for patients or their agents to voice their wishes about advanced directives forcefully.

Implications

The process of establishing appropriate care when death appears imminent is best conducted when the wishes of the patient are known ahead of time. It is the obligation of the patient's primary care physician to discuss possible scenarios, in the outpatient setting so that the physician knows the patient's wishes and can communicate them in intensive care situations. Advance directives facilitate this process, but such directives usually describe treatment choices in general terms and fall short of defining the specific situation.

The process of making appropriate decisions at the end of life is complex and often arduous. Although, in many circumstances, clear agreement exists concerning the ethical and legal basis for forgoing life support, physicians may still fail to understand the basis of sound ethical comportment and the law as it pertains to these issues. Physicians can no longer afford this luxury, and hospitals have an obligation to ensure that an effective ethics committee exists whose function includes the education of the medical and nursing staffs. Physicians cannot deliver appropriate clinical care without a firm understanding of the theory and application of medical ethics.

The definition and application of the concept of futility in the ICU will require broad debate in our pluralistic society. The process of applying futility judgments to decision making at the level of the individual, as well as to the appropriation of finite health care resources, still requires significant discussion. However, situations exist now in all ICUs that require appropriate decision making. Our recommendation is that the following definition be employed: a futile situation exists when ''treatment cannot within a reasonable probability cure, ameliorate, improve, or restore a quality of life that would be satisfactory to the patient'' (Quinn 1994).

Given this definition, an ongoing dialogue with the patient or health care proxy (usually a family member) can lead to appropriate decisions about continuation, advancement, withholding, or withdrawing of therapy. The situation is considerably clarified when advance directives and a formal process for forgoing therapy exist. When this approach is adopted, physician and patient or health care proxy most often arrive at a mutually acceptable plan. When disagreement develops, an ethics consultation should be initiated if this has not already been done. Every effort should be made to reach agreement on a therapeutic course. If an impasse remains despite such efforts, the physician has a severe dilemma. It is our opinion that the physician should choose a course of action that best protects the interests of the patient, guided by the definition of futility provided by Quinn (1994).

Conclusion

Many disease processes in critically ill patients have a high probability of death. Although this probability may approach 100% in many instances, it may often be lower, such as 60% to 80%. Despite our improved predictive abilities, not all outcomes can be anticipated with certainty. Formal policies for forgoing life support, such as advance directives, allow patients or health care proxies to forgo treatment under circumstances in which physicians think survival is unlikely. The situation is more complex when physicians believe that therapy is futile and the patient or health care proxy insists it be given. No formal ethics policy exists to guide physicians in this circumstance; the debate is evolving at present. The existence of value differences among health care workers and within the lay public render this task difficult. Ultimately, it appears likely that society and its institutions will be obligated to develop policy and guidelines that can be applied prospectively at the bedside in a just, equitable manner. Although physicians should be part of the debate, it is not their singular responsibility. If policies are developed asserting the right of the physician or hospital to curtail care at the end of life, their rationale should be expressly stated. We have offered a definition of futility and an approach to addressing end-of-life issues that we have found useful in providing a humane straightforward approach to dealing with difficult situations.

References

Asch, D.A., Hansen-Flaschen, J., and Lanken, P.N. 1995. Decisions to limit or continue life-sustaining treatment by critical care physicians in the United States: conflicts between physicians' practices and patients' wishes. *American Journal of Respiratory Disease and Critical Care Medicine* 151:288–92.

Haug, J.B., Harthug, S., Kalager, T., et al. 1994. Bloodstream infections at a Norwegian university hospital, 1974–1979 and 1988–1989. Changing etiology, clinical features, and outcome. *Clinical Infectious Diseases* 19:246–56.

Knaus, W.A., Draper, E.A., Wagner, D.P., and Zimmerman, J.E. 1985. Prognosis in acute organ-system failure. *Annals of Surgery* 202:685–93.

Landry, F.J., Parker, J.M., and Phillips, Y.Y. 1992. Outcome of cardiopulmonary resuscitation in the intensive care setting. *Archives of Internal Medicine* 152:2305–8.

Lemeshow, S., Teres, D., Klar, J., et al. 1993. Mortality probability models (MPM II) based on an international cohort of intensive care unit patients. *Journal of the American Medical Association* 270:2478–86.

Miranda, D.R. 1994. Quality of life after cardiopulmonary resuscitation. *Chest* 106:524–30.

Murphy, D.J., Burrows, D., Santilli, S., et al. 1994. The influence of the probability of survival on patients' preferences regarding cardiopulmonary resuscitation. *New England Journal of Medicine* 330:545–9.

Perl, T.M., Dvorak, L., Hwang, T., and Wenzel, R.P. 1995. Long-term survival and function after suspected gram-negative sepsis. *Journal of the American Medical Association* 274:338–45.

Peterson, M.W., Geist, L.J., Schwartz, D.A., et al. 1991. Outcome after cardiopulmonary resuscitation in a medical intensive care unit. *Chest* 100:168–74.

Quinn, J. B. 1994. Taking back their health care. *Newsweek* June 27, p. 36.

Rockwood, K., Noseworthy, T.W., Gibney, R.T.N., et al. 1993. One-year outcome of elderly and young patients admitted to intensive care units. *Critical Care Medicine* 21:687–91.

Sasse, K.C., Nauenberg, E., Long, A., et al. 1995. Long-term survival after intensive care unit admission with sepsis. *Critical Care Medicine* 23:1040–7.

Schapira, D.V., Studnicki, J., Bradham, D.D., et al. 1993. Intensive care, survival, and expense of treating critically ill cancer patients. *Journal of the American Medical Association* 269:783–6.

SUPPORT Principal Investigators. 1995. A controlled trial to improve care for seriously ill hospitalized patients. The Study to Understand Prognoses and Preferences for Outcomes and Risks of Treatments (SUPPORT). *Journal of the American Medical Association* 274:1591–8.

Tran, D.D., Groeneveld, A.B.J., van der Meulen, J., et al. 1990. Age, chronic disease, sepsis, organ system failure, and mortality in a medical intensive care unit. *Critical Care Medicine* 18:474–9.

Wachter, R.M., Luce, J.M., Safrin, S., et al. 1995. Cost and outcome of intensive care for patients with AIDS, *Pneumocystis carinii* pneumonia, and severe respiratory failure. *Journal of the American Medical Association* 273:230-5.

Yamani, M., Fleming, C., Brensilver, J.M., and Brandstetter, R.D. 1995. Using advance directives effectively in the intensive care unit. *Journal of Critical Illness* 10:465–73.

4

Physicians and medical futility: experience in the setting of general medical care

NORTON SPRITZ, M.D., J.D.

Futility – the doctor's dilemma

Patient autonomy, the dominating ethical principle that controls clinical decision making, evolved as a right of patients to be protected from inappropriate and unwanted application of life-extending medical technology. This principle reflects an ethical and legal consensus that serves to define the rights of patients and to set a standard against which physician and institutional actions can be judged.

Unfortunately, no comparable ethical consensus or body of law exists when the issue is not the right of patients to refuse treatment but instead is the limit to their rights to receive treatments. This issue appears when treatments under consideration have little chance to succeed or, on balance, provide little or no advantage to patients compared with the burdens that accompany their implementation. The term medical ''futility'' has come to encompass this group of problematic treatments.

In the clinical setting, the issue of futility can generally be described as follows: When is the value of a treatment or procedure sufficiently small or uncertain that it can be considered to be futile and, accordingly, the right of patients to choose it should be limited? Who decides that a medical treatment is futile, and what would be an equitable mechanism to establish and put into effect such determinations? A treatment may be considered futile either because the benefit of the treatment is unlikely to be realized or because, even if successful, there are serious limitations to the benefit to be achieved, as would be the case when the effect would be to continue a life in the permanently unconscious state.

Another aspect of medical futility relates to the burdensome nature of the procedures under question. A surrogate, for instance, may choose a treatment that would serve only to prolong a dying patient's life for a short time at the cost of undue pain or loss of personal dignity or both. Even in the absence of suffering by the patient, the treatment may be seen as excessive because its intrusive nature seems inappropriate for a short extension of life in a patient in whom there is no longer hope for control of the underlying fatal disease. The treatment may also be seen as excessive because its cost is disproportionate to its benefits, it deprives other patients of scarce resources, or it conflicts with broader societal values.

In considering these societal issues, it is important to separate limitations based on futility from those better classified as "rationing" (Jecker and Schneiderman 1992). The former is an individual and patient-based judgment, whereas the latter derives from a societal decision to limit individual access to certain medical resources in order to save money or other resources, and the ethical issue is one of distributive justice. As will be noted later, the distinction between these two processes may be ambiguous.

The risk of invoking futility to withhold care is that such decisions may be justified through a futility analysis that appears to focus on the patient's interest but is, in fact, driven by the interests of others. Fairness requires that patients and surrogates understand the degree to which decisions to withhold care with potentially problematic benefit reflect interests other than those of the patient. Debates concerning futility have not provided a consensus for a workable structure to deal with such issues. The absence of such a structure leaves the patient, surrogate, and caregivers to deal with these difficult issues in a way that is often inequitable and arbitrary. The futility issue has largely been framed as a struggle between physicians and patients for decisional power. The solutions offered have, unfortunately, tended to stake out one or the other extreme, neither of which is workable.

One position has been that the introduction of the issue of medical futility into clinical decision making is unwarranted. Those holding this point of view generally maintain that decisions that might be seen as futile do not differ fundamentally from standard clinical choices, and, accordingly, patient or surrogate control should not be limited (Truog, Brett, and Frader 1992). Although I agree that there is always a very strong presumption of patient autonomy, there are clearly instances, some depicted in this chapter, in which patient, professional, or societal considerations reasonably lead to limitations to the absolute right of patient determinism.

Some who recognize the validity of the concept of futility would limit its scope to circumstances in which the treatments under consideration produce no benefit, no matter how limited or problematic. This absolute definition of futility (physiologic futility), while maintaining semantic integrity, actually encompasses an extremely limited number of clinical circumstances and would not contribute to the development of ethical standards for limitation of care, as there is already consensus that there is no duty to provide treatment that lacks benefit.

Those holding the opposite point of view maintain that futility of certain medical measures is sufficiently evident that the underlying presumption of patient autonomy and control can be discarded (Schneiderman, Jecker, and Jonsen 1990). With this approach, when such circumstances have been identified, physicians would be empowered to decide against a procedure without the need for concurrence or even discussion with the patient or surrogate.

In recent analyses of this problem, several observers have noted that a workable approach to the issue of futility will have to represent a middle ground between the extremes of unlimited patient autonomy and absolute empowerment of physicians to designate certain clinical choices as futile (Truog 1995; Zawacki 1995). What seems to be envisioned is a process that strongly recognizes the right of patients to control decisions but also recognizes futility as a mechanism, rarely to be invoked, that would, with safeguards, place limitations on that right.

Another aspect of this evolving consensus requires that when futility is invoked to limit patient determination, the decision should not simply reflect the judgment of an individual physician but should, instead, result from some institutional or professional consensus (Nelson et al. 1994; Tomlinson and Czlonka 1995). Such a process may lead to generic designations of futility, such as a ruling that cardiopulmonary resuscitation (CPR) in all patients with a prognosis of less than one month to live is presumed to be futile. Alternatively, the designation of futility may result from institutional consideration of an individual case and apply directly to that patient.

Another important emerging consensus is that when an institutional process designates a treatment as futile, the designation serves only to establish a presumption against the treatment and need not serve as an absolute interdiction against its use in the individual instance. Such presumptions will, of course, shift the burden so that those who press for use of the treatment must define the special circumstances that warrant it. The process does, however, take into account that application of the principles of futility in the clinical arena is complex and subject to crucial individual considerations. Rather than limiting communication among patients, surrogates, and physicians, this process of an institutional definition of futility can lead to full and open discourse when properly applied. The patient or surrogate is informed that certain choices are considered to be futile on the basis of institutional consensus and that these choices will be offered to the patient only when individually justified.

This approach corrects the distortion in the decision-making process that occurs when untenable choices are presented to patients and surrogates as if they were reasonable possibilities. It also acts, appropriately, to transfer from the surrogate to the physician and institution some of the burdens that accompany a decision to withhold life-prolonging measures. Finally, knowledge of an institution's designations of futility may permit patients to be better able to select institutions whose policies are most in keeping with their own values and expectations.

In this chapter, I consider two clinical entities – chronic dialysis for end-stage kidney disease and the persistent vegetative state – as well as a single clinical encounter. Each of these examples depicts aspects of the issue of futility as it plays out in the clinical arena. In general, they reflect an attempt to find a reasonable middle ground between uninhibited patient autonomy and exclusion of patients and surrogates from the decision-making process that is consistent with the emerging consensus just discussed. These examples point out the importance of flexibility, communication among the involved parties, and individualization of the approach under varying clinical circumstances.

Chronic dialysis patients: two types of futility; two approaches

For chronic dialysis patients, continued life depends on adherence to an intense treatment program, but unlike patients requiring mechanical ventilation, for instance, dialysis patients spend most of their existence relatively unencumbered by their disease.

For patients in whom renal failure is temporary, dialysis permits survival until either renal function recovers or a healthy kidney is transplanted. Although the treatment of such patients raises important ethical issues, the patients whose only alternative to death is continuous long-term dialysis present the major challenge in relation to the issue of futility. For these patients, continued dialysis would seem to escape the issues that characterize questions of futility. Sufficient facilities to dialyze these patients are usually available, so that issues of scarce resources are not pertinent. General consensus that the resources necessary to provide dialysis are a valid expenditure of health care resources is expressed in the long-standing program of federal funding for this procedure. Questions of futility do, however, become pertinent as the quality of life of the dialysis patient diminishes. Such deterioration may result from renal failure per se or the occurrence of concomitant diseases that have a major impact on functional capacity, life expectancy, or both.

One special subset of patients in whom questions of futility arise when initiating or continuing dialysis are those with dementia. Dementia or some other forms of mental impairment may occur independently of the renal disease or may be related etiologically to the underlying renal disease but not be corrected by dialysis. Examples of the latter are common and include cerebral vascular disease with multiinfarct dementia as part of the generally accelerated atherosclerotic process that occurs in dialysis patients. In some instances, the patient makes the judgment that continued dialysis becomes futile as dementia develops. A decision may be made through an advanced directive prepared when the patient was in possession of decisional capacity. Ambiguity may arise when the directive is not put into effect because of the remote possibility that the demented state may improve or even disappear. Even more difficult questions may arise when the dementia is severe enough to preclude contemporaneous decisional capacity but is mild enough to allow for some meaningful life without apparent suffering.

Usually, there is no guiding advanced directive. Surrogates may be called on to decide on the basis of their impressions of the patient's wishes or their estimate of the patient's best interest whether it would be inappropriate to continue dialysis. If the patient's mental state leads him to interpret each dialysis as a threatening event that requires restraint or sedation or both, the decision to give up dialysis is most clearly in the patient's interest. In such a case, futility is being invoked through its least debatable and most clearly patient-directed mechanism – the procedure under question causes patient suffering not justifiable by its limited benefit.

Continuation of dialysis in the demented patient also brings into play the issue of the role and rights of the institution, other patients, and individual caregivers in such decisions. The staff of the dialysis unit often finds that dialysis imposed on an unwilling or resistant demented patient offends the staff's sense of professionalism and purpose of the unit. Theirs is a particularly distasteful role when the demented patient appears to be suffering. Such patients may also become a burden for other patients in the unit.

Several factors have led many dialysis units to adopt a general institutional policy that states that, in general, long-term dialysis is inappropriate for significantly demented patients. These factors include the burdens on other patients and staff, the communal nature of dialysis units that makes uniformity in treatment particularly important, and even though dialysis is financed through a federal program, the use of expensive resources to maintain severely demented patients, which raises issues of distributive justice.

As indicated, application of an institutional policy that generally considers dementia to preclude chronic dialysis need not be seen as an absolute edict but rather as a presumption against which each case must be measured. Cessation of dialysis need not be abrupt. It should be preceded by discussion, negotiation, and trials of dialysis to identify instances in which the dementia is reversible. There should be maximal discretion in dealing with ambiguous situations. An important element of such a policy is that it be equitably administered and that the policy of the dialysis program concerning demented patients be known to participants in the dialysis program at the time of their entry.

In contrast to patients with dementia, patients with intact decisional capacity may decide that the burdens of the dialysis procedure itself or the concomitant disability make continued dialysis inappropriate for the quality of life that it prolongs. Here, a decision to discontinue treatment should rest entirely under the patient's control.

When a chronic dialysis patient decides to discontinue dialysis, the physician's role is first to act in concert with the patient to identify correctable factors that might have led to this decision. This consideration may lead to bargaining for a delay in implementing the patient's wishes while such possibilities are explored. The physician and other members of the management team also must provide an unbiased but empathetic source of support. Finally, the dialysis team must not abandon a patient who has made the decision to forgo dialysis but must, instead, minimize suffering and maximize support as death approaches.

A single case that makes several points about futility

The management of a patient recently admitted to the medical service illustrates several important features of the futility issue as it may play out in individual clinical encounters. It illustrates, first, that the same set of factors can lead to different approaches, depending on the clinical context in which the problem occurs. Second, it demonstrates the importance of communication among all concerned and their participation in the decision-making process. Third, the case provides an instance in which, if communication and negotiations had failed, the patient and family might have made demands that the physician (with institutional review and support) would have been justified in rejecting. Finally, this case illustrates the overlap between the issue of futility, with its application to the individual patient, and distributive justice, in which the issue is societal in scope.

The patient experienced a massive life-threatening upper gastrointestinal hemorrhage, with no significant prior history. The bleeding resulted from a widespread malignant liver tumor that had infiltrated blood vessels in the stomach. Large quantities of transfused blood were necessary to prevent immediate death from exsanguination. Surgery, radiation, and chemotherapy were considered but were not reasonable options either for stopping the bleeding or for controlling the malignancy.

Despite the poor prognosis, it was decided to maintain the patient by vigorous blood replacement in order to give him and his loved ones the time necessary to understand, accept, and deal with the realities of his disease. Had this patient's hepatoma been diagnosed earlier and had this bleeding episode occurred as an event terminating the usual gradual downhill progression of the disease, the futility of intense and continued transfusion and the hopelessness of the clinical situation would have been confronted directly at the onset of the massive hemorrhage. For several days, the patient received sufficient blood to keep him relatively comfortable. He remained alert, and he and his relatives came to understand and accept the hopelessness of his illness. As agreed, we administered fewer transfusions while the treatment goal changed from extending life to preventing suffering. The patient and his family were informed that we expected a major vessel to erode soon, with resulting massive and immediately life-threatening hemorrhage. The medical staff, the patient, and his family understood that were this massive bleed to occur, we would not (and probably could not) administer blood at the rate necessary to prevent exsanguination.

In this case, the basis for invoking futility seemed clear. The benefit of intensive treatment of a massive bleed would be to extend life. Burdens included the short-lived period of intensive care treatment that would serve only to postpone death from the underlying malignant disease. The patient expressed his preference for a death from rapid exsanguination over death from the long-term effects of his malignant disease.

Some would argue that a decision to withhold transfusion as a scarce medical resource is not based on considerations of futility but rather reflects an issue of distributive justice. Although the patient rejected intensive and prolonged transfusion for personal reasons, the decision in this case illustrates the degree to which these two concepts overlap. Had the patient decided otherwise, his claim to the scarce resource would have been weakened by considerations that characterize the futility analysis. He would have lost out in competition for the scarce resource because its benefit under his clinical circumstances was problematic and limited – the essence of the futility analysis.

An important distinction must be made between limiting transfusions in circumstances such as this and decisions by physicians to limit care in the individual instance to decrease general health care costs. Unless such decisions are guided by societal policy that applies to all patients, they lead to inequitable restrictions on patient care that reflect the individual physician's bias.

Fortunately, in the great majority of instances, the patient or surrogate and those providing care come to a mutually acceptable course of action. As in this case, the agreement is based on communication that leads to understanding of the issues of importance to all concerned. If negotiation and explanation had failed to dissuade the family from a demand to administer massive transfusions indefinitely, we would have instituted a process to reject that demand, including consultation with the hospital ethics advisory committee.

Persistent vegetative state (PVS) and futility

A task force on PVS recently published an extensive review of PVS (The Multi-Society Task Force 1994). Their definition of PVS includes the following (1994:1499).

The vegetative state is a clinical condition of complete unawareness of the self and the environment, accompanied by sleep-wake cycles . . . in addition, patients in a vegetative state show no evidence of sustained, reproducible, purposeful, or voluntary behavioral responses to visual, auditory, tactile, or noxious stimuli; show no evidence of language comprehension or expression; have bowel and bladder incontinence. . . .

It is evident from this description, taken together with the intensity, intrusiveness, and expense of maintaining such lives, that PVS reflects a paradigm of the issues of medical futility. The effect of treatment in these patients can be defined as the extension of a life that is missing the basic characteristics associated with the human condition. Hope for recovery of some or all function depends to some degree on the age of the patient and the nature of the original brain injury. After three months of PVS, recovery in all categories of patients is quite unlikely, after six months, it is quite rare, and after twelve months, recovery is so rare that the task force was able to identify only six such patients, all of whom sustained permanent severe or moderate disability.

Beginning with the tragic case of Karen Quinlan (Angell 1991), PVS patients have served as the legal and ethical foundation of the right of patients or their surrogates to refuse treatment, even if that decision leads to death from the underlying diseases. The right to have life-sustaining treatments withheld or discontinued began with mechanical respiration in PVS patients. Subsequently, this right was extended to include the discontinuation of artificial feeding.

Decisions to discontinue life-sustaining treatments in PVS are fundamentally an application of medical futility. To many loved ones, continuation of these lives achieved no purpose but rather was a source of continuing pain. To those who care for PVS patients, the intense and prolonged effort to maintain their lives often seems out of proportion to any goal that is achieved and lacks the emotional reward associated with the care of responsive patients. At an institutional or societal level, expenditure of resources to extend these lives is hard to justify when compared with other medical needs.

The case of Helga Wanglie (Angell 1991), however, illustrates that even in PVS patients where the futility of indefinite prolongation of life seems to many to be at its clearest, discontinuation of treatment may violate strongly held beliefs. Mrs. Wanglie was an 87-year-old woman in a PVS for several months following a cerebral injury during surgery. The hospital informed her husband that in their view further support would be without benefit and indicated that they planned to discontinue her mechanical ventilation. Mr. Wanglie believed that this decision violated his wife's religious principles. The court rejected the hospital's assertion that Mr. Wanglie should be replaced as his wife's surrogate, and life support was continued until she died. This case illustrates that there are individual instances in which sincere, patient-centered arguments will support continued treatment even in clinical circumstances in which there is broad consensus that life support is futile.

It is crucial that we examine objectively the degree to which individual decisions to discontinue life support in PVS are driven by the patient's interests and the degree to which the determination of futility reflects primarily the interests of others. One can argue that the very inability of the PVS patient to perceive the environment – the cornerstone of the case for futility – also indicates that personal suffering by the patient cannot be a part of the burden–benefit analysis. In spite of the patient's contemporaneous inability to perceive pain or personal indignity, broader arguments have been put forth that define the PVS patient's interest in having treatment discontinued. These arguments, as put forth by Dworkin (1993), base the individual burden of continued life in PVS on an integrated view of patient autonomy and define a patient-centered rationale for discontinuing life support in a PVS patient. Dworkin puts it this way (1993:212).

Many people have a parallel reason for wanting to die if an unconscious vegetable life were all that remained. For some, this is an understandable worry about how they will be remembered, but for most, it is a more abstract and self-directed concern that their death, whatever else it is like, express their conviction that life had value because of what life made it possible for them to do and feel. They are horrified that their death might express, instead, the opposite idea, which they detest as a perversion: that mere biological life – just hanging on – has independent value.

Some PVS patients have advance directives that permit rejection of continued life in the PVS, and in those patients, discontinuation of life support is in direct accord with the principle of patient autonomy. Many persons without advance directives, possibly most, would have made that decision had they considered the issue when they possessed decisional capacity. It is, however, incorrect to attribute this point of view to all patients who do not have such a directive. Some, like the Wanglies, would define their interest to be the maintenance of life for as long as possible. Since limited recovery has been described even after prolonged periods of PVS, even this remote possibility may justify further maintenance of life in the absence of suffering.

Accordingly, although the argument for cessation of treatment is one that most of us may find compelling, the most honest analysis indicates that in the absence of advance directives or other clear evidence of the patient's wishes, the decision to discontinue life support in PVS is based most directly on interests other than those of the patient. These include the tremendous burdens that loved ones bear in seeing previously vital persons reduced to a vegetative state. Furthermore, continued support may strongly violate deeply held concepts of professional responsibility and the legitimate goals of patient care. Finally, institutional and societal interests in distributive justice in resource allocation constitute relevant considerations.

This argument bears emphasis, although not because it leads to the judgment that discontinuation of life support in PVS patients who have not made that prior choice is immoral or unethical. Instead, it points up the reality that individual autonomy, like any other important right, has its limitations and needs to be balanced against other considerations. It is important that we do not falsely invoke autonomy or attribute our view of the patient's interest to the patient when we make decisions that are based totally or even partially on interests of others. The more important issue is whether such decisions are being made in a fair way that allows for understanding and incorporation of the needs of patients and those who care about them.

The notion of individual dignity may play a role in institutional or societal decisions to terminate life support in PVS patients whose position is unknown. The concept of dignity indicates that the decision is not fundamentally inhumane and does not thoughtlessly negate the patient's rights. A dilemma remains, however, when the individual dignity argument has been rejected in favor of continued life either by the patient in advance directives or, more commonly, by those who speak for the patient. The decision to continue life may be based on religious grounds, as in the Wanglie family, or on the arguable best interest judgment that the patient who perceives no discomfort has nothing to lose by choosing continued life support, which allows for even the most remote possibility of partial recovery.

Two forces act together to minimize the number of instances in which there is direct conflict between demands on behalf of PVS patients and the concept of futility often held by their health care providers. Even with life support, PVS patients are subject to a high mortality, and there are relatively few long-term survivors. Surrogates for these patients generally agree that continued existence in a permanently unconscious state offends their sense of respect and dignity to which the patient is entitled.

It has been, in fact, the demand by families that life support be ended that has generally led to the involvement of the courts in this issue. This demand to terminate life-sustaining treatment underlies *Quinlan* and most of the cases that followed and has been the moral and legal underpinning of the right to refuse life-sustaining treatments.

Comparisons between PVS and brain death may be instructive. Brain-dead patients not only have lost their intellectual functions but also have sustained injury to the brainstem so that spontaneous respiration and other life-sustaining activities have ceased. Unlike for PVS, there are widely accepted criteria for the diagnosis of brain death and a broad legal and ethical consensus that these patients have died and that maintenance of life is improper or even illegal. Because of the variability in the clinical state and prognosis of PVS patients, it has been considerably more difficult to define a general policy. In individual situations, with institutional input when necessary, continued reevaluation of the patient's status and continued support of and communication with the responsible surrogate will generally lead to agreement. In situations like that of Helga Wanglie, however, when discontinuation of treatment conflicts with sincerely held religious beliefs, strong deference must be given such views, and continuation of support may be appropriate.

Conclusion

It is tempting to reject consideration of the issue of medical futility because its definition is elusive and its scope defies clear definition. To do so, however, is to leave a very difficult and important area of clinical care without consensus, standards, or guidelines. It ignores the reality that under certain circumstances, accepted treatments or procedures lack real benefit and, when instituted, may act against the patient's interest or that of others and also ignores the important fact that if demands for such treatment are made, the conflict may not be fairly resolved without some modification or limitation on patient autonomy.

Several factors lend urgency to the need to develop guiding principles against which individual or institutional actions, taken in the name of futility, can be judged. With or without guiding principles, decisions to withhold care on the basis of futility are made and instituted continually. In the absence of guiding principles, these decisions have a great potential for serious abuse. Individual decisions to withhold futile measures without guidelines are, at best, inequitable. Entitlement to treatments or protection from excessive treatment is based on the bias of the individual caregiver. At worst, without protective guidelines and a mechanism for review and broader debate, these decisions may be colored by discrimination against groups of patients or particular disease states.

References

Angell, M. 1991. The case of Helga Wanglie: a new kind of "right to die" case. *New England Journal of Medicine* 325:511–2.

Dworkin, R. 1993. *Life's Dominion*. New York: Knopf.

Jecker, N.S., and Schneiderman, L.J. 1992. Futility and rationing. *American Journal of Medicine* 92:189–96.

The Multi-Society Task Force on PVS. Medical aspects of the persistent vegetative state. 1994. *New England Journal of Medicine* 330:1499–1508, 1572–9.

Nelson, W., Durnan, J.R., Spritz, N., et al. 1994. Futility: the concept and its use. *Trends in Health Care, Law & Ethics* 9:19–26.

Schneiderman, L.J., Jecker, N.S., and Jonsen, A.R. 1990. Medical futility: its meaning and ethical implications. *Annals of Internal Medicine* 112:949–54.

Tomlinson, T., and Czlonka D. 1995. Futility and hospital policy. *Hastings Center Report* 25:(May–June)28–35.

Truog, R.D. Progress in the futility debate. 1995. *Journal of Clinical Ethics* 6:128–32.

Truog, R.D., Brett, A.S., and Frader, J. 1992. The problem with futility. *New England Journal of Medicine* 326:1560–4.

Zawacki, B.E. 1995. The "futility debate" and the management of Gordian knots. *Journal of Clinical Ethics.* 6:112–27.

5

Futility issues in pediatrics

JOEL E. FRADER, M.D., AND JON WATCHKO, M.D.

Many think that medical treatment for children is altogether different from that for adults. On the one hand, pediatrics seems to be about maintaining inherent good health through disease prevention, such as immunizations. On the other hand, we think of the obvious, even miraculous, advances in therapies for some childhood cancers (especially the most common, acute lymphocytic leukemia) and for disorders of the prematurely born. Unfortunately, pediatrics also has a less optimistic side. Some congenital anomalies, genetic disorders, and malignancies have not yet yielded to the press of modern medical science. Current technology and medical skill are unable to provide a reliably good outcome for very small preterm infants, certainly those born at 22 weeks of gestation or earlier, and a varying proportion of those born up to 26 weeks of gestation. The scourges of accidental injury, severe physical abuse, and AIDS continue to provide both enormous challenges and a depressing reminder of the limits of treatment.

Two features distinguish the futility confrontation in pediatrics faced by health care providers and the public from the confrontation in the rest of medicine. These are (1) our deeply held belief and hope that childhood should be different and that children should not die before some imaginary natural life span and (2) medical uncertainty in pediatrics, that is, the difficulty in predicting eventual outcomes, especially those pertaining to neurodevelopment. With these thoughts in mind, some issues in the debate over futile treatment in pediatrics are discussed.

Neonatal medicine

Most futility cases in pediatrics arise in neonatal care, particularly in the care of very premature infants. The history of futility disputes in this realm appears to parallel that in the rest of medicine generally and in intensive care in

48

particular. Thus, for years, some doctors seemed determined to press on with all treatments, often appearing indifferent to parental concerns about infant pain and suffering or the psychologic and economic impact on the family of continued treatment and the survival of a severely impaired child (Stinson and Stinson 1984; Harrison 1993). More recently, an increasing number of neonatologists, perhaps responding to the overzealousness of the past and sensitive to family concerns and desires, seem much more ready to recommend discontinuation of treatment. Ironically, some parents feel entitled to insist on continued mechanical ventilation and repeated resuscitations, expressing their religious beliefs of divine intervention on behalf of their child or their hostility and opposition to the willingness of physicians to forgo treatment.

Uncertainty

Decisions in medical treatment of the newborn have been hampered by difficulties in predicting outcomes for survivors. Recent consensus statements (Fetus and Newborn Committee 1994; Lantos et al. 1994) suggest wide agreement that those born before 22 completed weeks of gestation have no chance of survival and that treatment decisions regarding pregnant women and their fetuses at that age should depend entirely on factors relevant to the mother (e.g., cesarean section should be performed only for maternal indications). After birth, such babies should receive comfort care alone. Between 22 and 26 completed weeks of gestation, the likelihood of survival and the probability of survival without major handicap (e.g., intellectual deficit, neurosensory impairment, chronic lung disease) increase with each week, if not each day. Even so, at 23 to 24 weeks of gestation, mortality and significant neonatal morbidity are commonplace, so that approximately 90% of infants born at 23 weeks gestation and approximately 65% of infants born at 24 weeks gestation will die or have long-term adverse neurodevelopmental sequelae (Allen, Donohue, and Dusman 1993). As a result, for these infants, many in North America recommend deference to parental wishes about how actively to apply the measures available in newborn intensive care facilities. In Britain, where more decision-making authority remains in the hands of physicians, a survey of neonatal units revealed "wide variations in clinical practice" regarding decisions to ventilate very low birth weight babies (Day and Primhak 1993).

It can thus be inferred that there are no clear statistical or moral norms to provide guidance to physicians or family members in an individual case. Outcome varies with maternal health (and perhaps prenatal care), gestational age, biologic factors specific to the particular baby, the resources at hand when an infant is born (for example, the availability of surfactant to treat the lungs of premature infants deficient in this substance), the skill of the particular health care providers [outcome varies from one intensive care nursery to another, even after attempting to adjust for different populations of infants (Hack et al. 1994)], and the convictions and commitments of those participating in treatment decisions. Moreover, in the absence of absolute statistical certainty, that is, a 0 or 100% probability of a particular outcome, there will be disagreement about the probability of a given result that justifies initiating, continuing, or stopping treatment (Lantos et al. 1989; Fischer and Stevenson 1987; Truog, Brett, and Frader 1992).

Publicized cases illustrate this point. One case involved the premature infant of a physician and his wife in Michigan. Apparently, the father (a dermatologist), his spouse, and some of the involved medical personnel discussed what to do when Mrs. Messinger went into preterm labor. The parents-to-be expressed the view that the pregnancy had not progressed sufficiently far to justify resuscitation or similar intervention in the delivery room. Those attending the delivery either did not accept or know of the parents' views, and the infant was treated vigorously, taken to the neonatal intensive care unit (NICU), and provided with mechanical ventilation. Angered by these events and convinced that treatment was futile, the father went to the NICU and disconnected the infant from life support, ensuring death. The father was later prosecuted for a criminal offense but was acquitted by a jury.

By contrast, another preterm infant, born in Washington state, became the object of heated attention when, after a few weeks of very active treatment, he developed important complications – neurologic injury, gastrointestinal obstruction, and kidney failure. The hospital physicians declared that further therapy was inappropriate. Ryan Nguyen's parents refused to accept this judgment and obtained legal counsel to support their press for continued therapy. Learning of the dispute from the media, physicians at another hospital in the region contacted the family and accepted the child for the interventions that the parents desired.

These cases illustrate the fundamentally different perspectives and values brought to bear when futility debates arise. We find little agreement on medical, religious, philosophical, economic, or procedural grounds for deciding whether or not such infants deserve the full technical measure that neonatal care can provide. The recent literature suggests, however, that approximately 85% of NICU deaths occur following a decision to limit or withdraw life-sustaining medical treatment (Campbell, Lloyd, and Duffty 1988; Ryan et al.

1993; Cook and Watchko 1996). Most of these decisions involve agreement between health care professionals and parents.

Legality

No discussion of futility in neonatal care can ignore the unprecedented and controversial attempt of U.S. federal legislation to profoundly affect the practice of medicine. In brief, the 1984 amendments to the Child Abuse and Neglect Law resulted from a prolonged legal and political battle following the planned death of an infant, born in 1982 in Indiana, with Down syndrome (trisomy 21) and esophageal atresia. That death initially resulted in regulatory intervention by the Department of Health and Human Services (DHHS) of the Reagan administration. They alleged that the physicians violated the Rehabilitation Act of 1973, meant to prevent discrimination against the disabled. These regulations were voided by federal court action. Subsequently, Congress amended existing federal legislation that focused on child abuse and neglect. Supported by a coalition of medical and advocacy groups, federal lawmakers created a new category of child abuse, "medical neglect," whereby "handicapped" infants were expected to receive all available treatment unless three exceptions applied.

These exceptions allow doctors to withhold or withdraw treatment if they determine (1) that the infant in question is "chronically and irreversibly comatose," or if treatment would be (2) "futile in terms of . . . survival" or (3) "virtually futile . . . and . . . inhumane." In no case may "appropriate nutrition, hydration, and medication" be withheld or withdrawn. The law, of course, does not define any of the key words, especially "futile," "inhumane," and "appropriate" (Pub. L. 98-457 1984). Interpretive guidelines from DHHS in subsequent implementing regulations make it clear that those issuing the rules intended that quality of life considerations not be taken into account in determining how to treat infants covered by the law. The final regulations adopted after the DHHS received over 100,000 comments offer little guidance beyond the language of the statute. Statistical determinations of futility are not discussed in either the law or the regulations. Thus, there is no clear basis for knowing when federal law might recognize an exception to the requirements for all-out treatment.

The impact of the legislation and regulations has been difficult to gauge. Many neonatologists and pediatricians appear not to recognize that the law has little or no direct applicability to them, as outlined subsequently. The law requires that states receiving federal funds for child abuse and neglect programs use child protective systems to provide for reporting and investigating allegations of medical neglect of handicapped infants. Each state must have the means to ensure that endangered infants receive treatment. The only means of enforcement under the law is loss of federal funding for the state's child abuse program. The federal law provides no method to hold parents, physicians, or health care institutions accountable for violations of its provisions. Nevertheless, at least one survey (Kopelman, Irons, and Kopelman 1988) indicated that physicians caring for "imperiled" newborns think that their clinical judgment and freedom to make decisions with parents have been unduly altered. Thus, despite the determination that futile treatment need not be provided to newborns, it seems that continuing uncertainty, confusion, and fear about what actually constitutes futile treatment may result in less forgoing of life support.

Older children

Futility cases in pediatrics beyond the newborn period appear to be fairly similar to cases in adult medicine. However, our hopes and aspirations for children seem to make it more difficult for everyone involved to accept that medical science has nothing more to offer a sick or injured child. That some unfortunate children have not had the opportunity to live out a full life makes the acceptance of fatal disorders more tragic. Some even have particular religious views that embody a belief that children must not be allowed to die, if at all possible, before having lived to the end of a natural life span. In one recent case, members of an evangelical Christian church insisted on caring for the ventilated body of a brain-dead teenager at home for months, saying they believed that God would not permit the death of one so young.

The medical literature and the media have highlighted a number of cases of futility disputes about children. One highly publicized case in Florida involved a child who became brain dead after suffering complications of diabetes. The child's family refused to accept an apparently standard medical diagnosis of brain death. When discussions with family members broke down, officials from a Sarasota hospital sought court approval of a decision to stop artificial support. Although the court affirmed that physicians in Florida could indeed declare a person dead despite surrogate dissent, it did not specifically authorize stopping mechanical ventilation or artificial hydration. Frustrated, the hospital arranged for home care of the brain-dead child at the hospital's expense (the family's insurance coverage had been exceeded).

Other cases have involved children with AIDS, degenerative neurologic conditions, severe brain injury following child abuse, severe encephalopathy with recurrent respiratory failure, and lethal lung disease. The case of Baby K, born and resuscitated in the delivery room according to the mother's wishes after prenatal ultrasound diagnosis of anencephaly, included a long legal battle that ended in a federal appeals court.

Problems with decision making

In the cases involving children that have been adjudicated, the courts generally have not supported physician or hospital requests for authority to make unilateral medical decisions against the wishes of parents. If anything is clear in the futility wars over children, it is that doctors and health care organizations in the United States cannot count on the legal system to help them when parents or other guardians dissent from the medical recommendations. Yet, for the most part, this is precisely what the debate over futility determinations has been about – the legitimacy of unilateral, that is, medical, decision making.

In a series of three articles, Paris et al. (Paris, Crone, and Reardon 1990, 1991; Paris et al. 1993) argued that traditional medical ethics, reinforced in the public discussion reflected in the report of the President's Commission (1981), holds that health care providers need not offer or employ measures beyond those of the standard of care or strongly held personal beliefs. Extensive consideration of how we should construe any given standard of care or how we should regard the role of the personal conscience of the professional in medical situations exceeds the scope of this discussion. Nevertheless, it is worth noting that legal standards of care are often decided by juries, although informed by medical experts – that is, there is an important public nonmedical component to the notion of standard of care. Also, we sometimes constrain physician behavior with respect to personal beliefs. Despite strong personal views, doctors may not simply override the wishes of patients whenever they wish. For example, physicians caring for a competent patient who accepts the antitransfusion doctrine of the Jehovah's Witnesses may not employ blood products even to save the patient's life.

In short, there is little consensus on precisely what grounds justify rejecting the values that parents or other surrogates bring to the medical arena. Despite the claims of Paris et al. (1990, 1991), even appeals to the well-worn concept of the best interests of the child beg the questions of who determines those interests and on what basis. We have no medical, social, cultural, or moral gold standard for deciding what is best for any child who cannot make that determination for himself or herself.

Resource allocation and futility

Limited resources for medical care have also been cited by many authors as a justification for allowing physicians to determine when treatment is futile and to stop treatment so judged. Again, we cannot review here all the arguments for and against bedside economic determinations. What seems evident, however, is that health care rationing, if permitted, should be explicit. We should not allow claims of medical futility to mask decisions that really have cost savings as their principal aim. Although few of us would celebrate the hundreds of thousands of dollars spent on long-term mechanical ventilation for anencephalic children, brain-dead bodies, or other patients for whom there seems to be no benefit, such expenditures are most likely small compared with unnecessary neuroimaging for complaints of headache, inappropriate antibiotic prescriptions for self-limited viral infections, and the many other everyday excesses of modern American medicine. We need rational public discourse and resultant reasonable policy based on widespread community agreement.

Some hospitals, for example, the Children's Hospital in San Diego, California, have begun to formulate and disseminate policies on futile treatment. These may permit physicians, often with a required concurring second medical opinion, to declare treatment futile and refuse to provide or continue such therapy. Some policies require consultation with or agreement by an institutional ethics committee. If families then take no further action, attending physicians may indeed withhold or withdraw therapy. These policies seem to place an especially high burden on families from poor and minority communities with fewer resources and less political power to challenge doctors and hospitals.

Besides the problem of inequities in economic and social status, decisions made by ethics committees raise another concern, that of institutional (economic) self-interest. Although futility cases in pediatrics probably represent a tiny fraction of the overall health care budget spent on children, any given case may represent a substantial economic burden for a particular hospital. One can well imagine that institutional managers or others with interests tied to the welfare of a hospital would bring substantial explicit or covert pressure on ethics committee members to accept a claim of medical futility. As capitated arrangements, with their limited budgets, become more common, such conflicts of interest will become even more important. The multidisciplinary nature of an ethics committee will provide little protection from these conflicts of interest, as virtually all members of the group will likely either be institutional employees or have a strong economic connection to the organization.

Professional–family interaction

One of the most worrisome aspects of the futility debate concerns the way these conflicts may play themselves out. The report by Paris et al. (1993) of refusal to prolong the use of extracorporeal membrane oxygenation (ECMO) for a 5-year-old boy may provide an instructive example. The authors describe the case of an unfortunate boy who suffered severe trauma followed by respiratory failure, probably resulting from adult-type respiratory distress syndrome. ECMO was started as a ''last-stage heroic measure,'' and the family apparently ''agreed to a two-week trial'' of the treatment in the hope of lung recovery. During those weeks, renal failure ensued and liver dysfunction developed. Attempts at conventional respiratory support failed. As the trial period ended, the parents objected to withdrawing ECMO, knowing that the child would die without it. After obtaining support from an ethics committee, the treating physicians told the protesting family when ECMO would be stopped. The family was present when the treatment was withdrawn and the boy died.

What is missing from the report of this case is precisely what we must not allow to happen when doctors decide that treatment is futile. We have no evidence of the necessary personal interaction with the family that should lead up to treatment withdrawal. We can find nothing about the inevitable parental guilt that might well inhibit family members from agreeing to the end of therapy. We can find no discussion of the family's personal beliefs that might influence their thinking about termination of treatment, nor can we find anything about the compassionate support needed by grieving families that should be provided by members of the treatment team in such cases. We do not know whether these elements of care occurred in this case or not, as they do not appear in the published report. However, failure to mention these caring components may well mirror their lack of importance in much of today's medical care.

The usual litany of reasons for inadequate interaction between family members and health care providers includes their social, economic, and cultural differences, lack of time that busy professionals have for nontechnical matters, and inadequate education about interactive skills and medical ethics. One also has to worry that inadequate interaction represents a kind of backlash against the movement that secured patient or family autonomy in medical decision making in the last 25 years. Physicians may feel disenfranchised and use futility as a lever in the struggle for empowerment in medical decisions. Some doctors may have become alienated from themselves, as well as from their patients and loved ones, when they became technical superspecialists, and they may want to regain a measure of lost moral authority. Their attempts to truncate and trump medical decisions through futility claims, however, do not seem to be the best way to return to a trusted position in the doctor–patient–family relationship.

Conclusion

The debate over medical futility in pediatrics has some distinctive features, namely, the meaning that children have for most of us and the relatively high degree of medical uncertainty that pertains to some cases, especially those involving neonates. In addition, some futility cases appear to result from attempts to improve the allocation of medical resources. Finally, for some, attempts to impose medical decisions based on futility determinations may represent a reaction to wholesale failures of relationships in today's impersonal subspecialty-oriented medicine.

None of these problems has a simple or straightforward solution. Physicians need to do a much better job of educating families about the limitations of medicine, especially our restricted prognostic capabilities and the lack of relationship between the media's miracle-filled medicine and the realities of everyday practice. Medical education could do more to help doctors improve their communication skills and gain a genuine understanding of and tolerance for the belief systems of others. Public policy may press for better communication, as New Jersey law arguably provides when it permits personal objections to brain death determinations.

Physicians must enter, if not lead, a public debate about medical resources and rationing policies. Insistence on unilateral decision making seems not only wrongheaded (after all, it is not clear that there is a morality exclusive to the practice of medicine) but a prescription for widening the already substantial gulf between medical professionals and those who use the scientific health care system.

References

Allen, M.C., Donohue, P.K., and Dusman, A.E. 1993. The limit of viability – neonatal outcome of infants born at 22 to 25 weeks' gestation. *New England Journal of Medicine* 329:1597–601.

Campbell, A.G.M., Lloyd, D.J., and Duffty, P. 1988. Treatment dilemmas in neonatal care: who should survive and who should decide? *Annals of the New York Academy of Sciences* 530:92–103.

Cook, L.A., and Watchko, J.F. 1996. Decision-making for the critically ill neonate near the end of life. *Journal of Perinatology*16:133–6.

Day, C., and Primhak, R.A. 1993. Current practices in neonatal intensive care in the United Kingdom. *British Medical Journal* 307:362.

Fetus and Newborn Committee, Canadian Paediatric Society and Maternal-Fetal Medicine Committee, Society of Obstetricians and Gynaecologists of Canada. 1994. Management of the woman with threatened birth of an infant of extremely low gestational age. *Canadian Medical Association Journal* 151:547–53.

Fischer, A.F., and Stevenson, D.K. 1987. The consequences of uncertainty: an empirical approach to medical decision making in neonatal intensive care. *Journal of the American Medical Association* 258:1929–31.

Hack, M., Taylor, H. G., Klein, N., et al. 1994. School-age outcomes in children with birth weights under 750 g. *New England Journal of Medicine* 331:753–9.

Harrison, H. 1993. The principles for family-centered neonatal care. *Pediatrics* 92:643–50.

Kopelman, L.M., Irons, T.G., and Kopelman, A.E. 1988. Neonatologists judge the "Baby Doe" regulations. *New England Journal of Medicine* 318:677–83.

Lantos, J.D., Singer, P.A., Walker, R.M., et al. 1989. The illusion of futility in clinical practice. *American Journal of Medicine* 87:81–4.

Lantos, J.D., Tyson, J.E., Allen, A., et al. 1994. Withholding and withdrawing life sustaining treatment in neonatal intensive care: issues for the 1990s. *Archives of Disease in Childhood* 71:F218–23.

Paris, J.J., Crone, R.K., and Reardon, F. 1990. Physicians' refusal of requested treatment: the case of Baby L. *New England Journal of Medicine* 322:1012–15.

Paris, J.J., Crone, R.K., and Reardon, F. 1991. Ethical context for physician refusal of requested treatment. *Journal of Perinatology* 11:273–5.

Paris, J.J., Schreiber, M.D., Statter, M., et al. 1993. Beyond autonomy – physicians' refusal to use life-prolonging extra-corporeal membrane oxygenation. *New England Journal of Medicine* 329:354–7.

President's Commission for the Study of Ethical Problems in Medicine and Biomedical and Behavioral Research. 1981. *Defining Death: Medical, Legal and Ethical Issues in the Definition of Death*. Washington, DC: Government Printing Office.

Ryan, C.A., Byrne, P., Kuhn, S., and Tyebkhan J. 1993. No resuscitation and withdrawal of therapy in a neonatal and a pediatric intensive care unit in Canada. *Journal of Pediatrics* 123:534–8.

Stinson, A., and Stinson, P. 1984. *The Long Dying of Baby Andrew*. New York: Atlantic Monthly Press.

Truog, R.D., Brett, A.S., and Frader, J. 1992. The problem with futility. *New England Journal of Medicine* 326:1560–4.

Statutes and cases

1984 Amendments to the Child Abuse Prevention and Treatment Act. Pub. L. 98–457.

6

Medical futility: a nursing home perspective

ELLEN KNAPIK BARTOLDUS, M.S.W.

"The term medical futility has become a shorthand way to describe a situation in which the patient demands and the physician objects to the provision of certain medical treatment on the ground that the treatment will provide no medical benefit to the patient" (Daar 1995:221). The debate on the issue of medical futility has focused primarily on the care and treatment provided in the acute care setting. But questions about how medical futility decisions are reached also have profound implications for nursing homes, the institutions created to care for the oldest and most vulnerable of our society.

Discussion of what may be considered medically futile treatment goes to the heart of what it means to provide care and treatment for the dependent elderly, how we define and value life, and how we view the role of medical technology. These considerations define the role of the nursing home as a care-giving institution. How do we as a society create the kind of environment that will allow us to number our days in comfort and dignity while dealing with the difficult decisions that medical technology has foisted upon us? A number of factors may influence the manner in which the issue of medical futility is explored and resolved in the nursing home.

The role of nursing homes

As institutions, nursing homes are challenged to both care and cure. Mandated under the Federal Omnibus Budget Reconciliation Act (OBRA) of 1987, as well as state regulations, to assist their residents in reaching and maintaining their highest functional level, the emphasis on rehabilitative services, optimal functioning, and encouragement of residents to maintain their past interests and involvements has become central to developing a plan of care for all nursing home residents. Individual autonomy has become an important focus of our approach to nursing home life, and residents are expected to maintain their independence and former lifestyles to the extent possible. This emphasis may reflect values deeply held within American society: rugged individualism and self-sufficiency. As nursing homes struggle to help residents maintain their independence, however, they are also challenged to create a place of authentic and skillful care for those who can no longer care for themselves. They are institutions that are called on to offer medical, nursing, and residential services to a population whose members suffer declining physical or mental function or both, and increasingly withdraw from the outside world. Many residents will live out their days in a nursing home, where the residential and social aspects of life encounter the need for medical services. In fact, the medical aspects often become the central focus. This dual role, caring and curing, differentiates nursing homes from the acute care setting and presents a different context for decisions regarding medical futility.

Concerns about medical treatment

Although challenged to fulfill this dual mandate, nursing homes are stringently regulated at federal, state, and local levels in ways that hospitals are not. Because of the strong focus on the state survey process, whose purpose is to ensure regulatory compliance, administrators and nursing directors experience considerable anxiety concerning options for medical decision making by or on behalf of critically ill residents (Kapp 1990:286). Often, the responsible persons in nursing homes prefer to avoid the need to confront questions about medically futile treatment by transferring a resident to an acute care setting for evaluation and treatment. This may place the resident at a serious disadvantage because discussions about his or her care are now being made among strangers.

It is unusual for a physician in a nursing home to be asked to provide medical treatment that a resident or family member deems futile. In the absence of an advance directive to the contrary, a physician may feel compelled either by law or by practice to recommend a medical treatment that may be seen as having questionable benefit to the resident. "Benefit" is a value-laden term that can be interpreted in a variety of ways. Schneiderman (1994: 884) postulates that

the physicians's charge is to provide not merely an *effect* upon some part of the body, but a *benefit* to the patient as a whole. Medicine today has the capacity to achieve a multitude of effects. . . . none of these effects is a benefit unless the patient has, at the very least, the capacity to appreciate it, . . . an effect is not a benefit if it cannot

enable the patient to achieve, at a minimum, life goals other than complete "preoccupation" . . . with the patient's illness and treatment.

As in the acute care setting, determination of the benefit of a particular
treatment to a patient is often difficult. In the nursing home, the special
relationships often established between staff and residents may make the issue
more controversial. Life in a nursing home has many dimensions. It is a web
of interrelationships in which people are caring and being cared for. Relationships between residents and staff tend to be long term. Over time, as staff
and residents get to know one another's stories, histories, families, and ways
of looking at the world, strong attachments often develop. Sometimes, members of the direct care staff feel as if they understand the resident better than
anyone else. We ask this staff, particularly the nursing assistants who have
the most frequent and intimate contact with the resident, to meet residents'
needs in a personal and individualized fashion, yet we often fail to acknowledge the power of these relationships as we explore the ways in which treatment decisions are made. In working through these issues with staff, it is
important to distinguish between futile medical treatment and futile care. The
word "futile" implies a sense of hopelessness, a sense that a specific action
is in vain. Although a particular medical treatment may be considered to
produce no benefit to the resident, staff often needs to be reassured that their
caring is never futile, never in vain. The decision to forgo a particular treatment must never be confused with abandoning the resident.

The concern about resident abandonment may also reflect the cultural attitudes and beliefs of some nursing home staff. Many nurses and nursing
assistants come from cultures in which nursing homes, as we know them, do
not exist. The elderly are cared for within the family and extended family
structures. Some nursing assistants have confided, "I would never place my
mother in a nursing home," even though they know that they provide excellent care. Others have indicated a belief that once a family places a resident
in a nursing home, this act of abandonment reduces a family's right to be
involved in decision making about their relative's care. Sometimes, a staff
member may view herself as the one person who refuses to abandon a resident and may feel that withholding or withdrawing a particular medical treatment is tantamount to "standing by and letting someone die."

Nowhere is this more evident than in relation to decisions about withholding or withdrawing artificial nutrition and hydration. "The fact that there is
a legal consensus about the propriety of foregoing artificial nutrition and
hydration does not mean that it is well accepted. And in no health care setting
is it so difficult to withhold or withdraw feeding tubes as in nursing homes"

(Maisel 1995:618). Since food and water are basic to human survival, the decision to withhold or withdraw a feeding tube may be seen not as the withholding of a medical treatment but rather as the denial of basic human care.

Some of the difficulty surrounding the issue of withdrawing artificial nutrition and hydration lies in the manner in which the decisions are made and the capacity of the resident to make his or her wishes known. When residents are able to choose, the decision to withhold artificial nutrition and hydration may be more comfortable for staff. One nurse discussed her reaction to a long-time resident's refusal of tube feeding.

I was really hurt and saddened by Ruth's decision and couldn't understand why she didn't want to accept the tube feeding and continue to fight. I hated the thought of her "starving to death," but once we were able to talk about it, I realized that she had made her choice and that she was comfortable with it. I felt able to respect that choice and take care of her until she died here at home with us.

The situation becomes more difficult when residents are unable to make their wishes known directly or through a health care proxy or some other form of advance directive. Some nursing home staff believe that if no advance directive exists, there is a moral and legal obligation to do everything medically possible for the resident.

Advance directives

Advance directives play an important role in the discussion of medical futility. With the passage of the 1991 Patient Self-Determination Act, nursing homes were mandated by law to discuss the issue of advance directives with all residents on admission. Advance directives create a mechanism by which individuals can make their wishes known about particular medical treatments should they become incapable of making an informed decision in the future. Advance directives do not offer much guidance, however, in a discussion of medical futility. The reality is that advance directives are geared toward helping patients refuse rather than secure treatment.

The ongoing nature of the relationship between staff and residents places nursing homes in a unique position to assist residents in making their wishes known through advance directives. The way in which the issue is approached is critical. Frequently, when residents are asked about their interest in creating advance directives, they are presented with a series of hypothetical situations and the possible medical interventions they may or may not want under particular circumstances. Rather than approaching the development of advance directives as a list of acceptable or nonacceptable medical interventions, we might (Moody 1992:65)

think of advance directives as occasions for communication, not as a means of definitely setting treatment decisions. . . . (T)he very act of writing a living will or making a power of attorney provides an occasion for getting all concerned parties – patient, family members, health care professionals – to talk with one another about treatment decisions. Ambivalence and confusion may still remain, but the activity of communication fulfills its purpose.

This act of communication offers an opportunity to see residents within the context of their larger life experience and, in doing so, decreases the possibility of conflict around medically futile treatment. Conversations with the resident can focus on how he or she would choose to spend the remaining years of life. What gives life meaning to this resident? What tasks and dreams are still unfulfilled, and what kind of care can we offer that might facilitate their accomplishment? Finally, how does this resident view dependency on specific medical treatments to maintain life, and are there circumstances under which the resident might choose to forgo treatment? Communication on this level would help the resident build trust not only in the individual chosen as the health care proxy but also in the physician and the nursing home as a whole. The challenge to the nursing home community is to create a safe place where these discussions can occur and to develop new methods to facilitate communication around these profound issues.

Dementia and decision making

Whereas advance directives may be helpful for some nursing home residents, others may not be capable of communicating their wishes because of Alzheimer's disease or other forms of advanced dementia. Nursing homes must seek ways to understand the reality of a demented resident and encourage participation in the decision-making process to the extent possible. How can we best approximate the values and desires of a demented resident at this stage of life? Dresser and Whitehouse (1994:7) state

The vast majority of dementia patients have an experiential world. Unlike Nancy Cruzan and Karen Quinlan, most dementia patients are subjects with their own thoughts, perceptions, emotions and perspectives. These patients themselves are affected by the medical interventions they receive – they subjectively experience the consequences of the treatment decisions made on their behalf. Yet the subjectivity of the dementia patient is often overlooked. The increasing number of treatment dilemmas involving patients with dementia challenges clinicians and policy makers to develop a more principled approach to evaluating "what it is like" to be a particular patient whose treatment is at issue.

The long-term commitment of nursing homes to residents, particularly those with dementia, places them in an excellent position to explore and develop new approaches to this issue.

Conclusion

The key to providing compassionate care lies in the ability of the nursing home to create a bond with the resident and significant others in which there is truth telling, open communication, confidence, and the unfailing belief that the resident is at the center of all decisions involving personal care. When this bond can be developed and the resident has confidence in the physician and caregiving staff, issues of medical futility become less significant. Nursing homes must begin to develop not a medicine of strangers but rather a medicine of intimates. According to Siegler (1992:68)

[I]n relations among strangers, rules and procedures become very important, and control rather than trust is dominant. Strangers do not know each other well enough to have mutual trust. Thus, in the absence of intimate knowledge or of shared values, strangers resort to rules and procedures to establish control. By contrast, in relations of intimacy, all parties know each other very well and often share values or at least know which values they do not share. In such relations, formal rules and procedures, backed by sanctions, may not be necessary; they may even be detrimental to the relationships. In relations of intimacy, trust rather than control is dominant. Trust means confidence in and reliance upon the other party to act in accord with moral principles and rules.

The nursing home community has much to offer to the current debate about medical futility. In a true medicine of intimates, the futility debate goes away. As patients trust their physicians and the staff caring for them, the communication process would permit consensus, rather than conflict, to determine medical futility. Basic to any discussion of the issue is our willingness to see aging not as a medical problem to be solved but as part of the life process. Medical science has yet to conquer death, and death is an inevitable outcome of the aging process. Our denial of our own mortality often creates conflict around issues of medical futility. Although education about advance directives and their creation may be helpful, and we must explore new ways to promote ethical decision making for those suffering from dementia, our real challenge is to create within the nursing home a community based on trust and, most important, compassion. "Compassion is the quality of the human heart that makes it possible for people of very different ages and life styles to meet each other and form community'' (Nouwen and Gaffney 1976:114). It is within the creative tension of this community that we can better understand what it means to provide care for the elderly and face the issue of medical futility with openness and integrity.

References

Daar, J.F. 1995. Medical futility and implications for physician autonomy. *American Journal of Law and Medicine* 21:221–40.

Dresser, R., and Whitehouse, P.J. 1994. The incompetent patient on the slippery slope. *Hastings Center Report* 24(July–August):6–12.

Kapp, M. 1990. State of the law: nursing homes. *Law, Medicine and Health Care* 18:282–9.

Maisel, A. 1995. *The Right to Die*, 2nd ed. New York: Wiley, vol. 1.

Moody, H.R. 1992. *Ethics in an Aging Society*. Baltimore: Johns Hopkins Press.

Nouwen, H.J.M., and Gaffney, W.J. 1976. *Aging: The Fulfillment of Life*. New York: Doubleday.

Schneiderman, L.J. 1994. The futility debate: effective versus beneficial intervention. *Journal of the American Geriatrics Society* 42:883–6.

Siegler, M. 1992. A medicine of strangers or a medicine of intimates: the two legacies of Karen Ann Quinlan. *Second Opinion* 17(4):64–8.

7

Alternative medicine and medical futility

JOSEPH J. JACOBS, M.D., M.B.A.

He who conceals his disease cannot expect to be cured.
(Ethiopian proverb)

Many of us, especially those of us trained in modern medicine, believe in the primacy of science and its ability to find a cure for what ails us. That belief is shaken by the prevalence of chronic or recurrent debilitating diseases and by death itself. The wish for something now and for something more effective than what science offers leads in the direction of alternative medicine. Uncertainty as to what is effective is heightened by the fact that many conditions other than terminal illness have a psychologic component and may be improved by alternative therapy; low back pain and insomnia are good examples.

Eisenberg et al. (1993) defined alternative medicine as "medical interventions not widely taught at U.S. medical schools or generally available at U.S. hospitals." Cassileth et al. (1984) found that cancer patients who used alternative treatments were better educated than patients who used only conventional therapy. These authors concluded that there was a selective bias toward educated patients because they have the financial, educational, and personal resources to learn about these therapies and to provide support for their families during this time. Lerner and Kennedy (1992) reported similar characteristics. The better educated have also been taught not to take authority at face value.

The unrealistic expectations of individuals who are desperate to find a solution to a pressing clinical need are well illustrated by a call I received while I was Director of the Office of Alternative Medicine at the National Institutes of Health. I was awakened around 3:00 a.m. one Saturday by a telephone call from a woman whose mother was in a coma from a stroke. She mistakenly thought that I was a traditional Native American healer and asked if I could come to Ohio to pray for her mother. Needless to say, I was startled by this request. I gently informed her that I did not have this power and that I understood her pain and frustration. I asked her to call me in the office on the following Monday. Although she never called, I could share the woman's feeling of desperation and understand her willingness to reach out even to something as relatively unorthodox as a Native American healing ceremony to help to save her mother.

How often is alternative therapy used for fatal illnesses? According to Eisenberg et al. (1993), 34% of a random sample of adults reported using alternative medicine for cancer. Cassileth et al. (1984) found that 13% of patients at the University of Pennsylvania Cancer Center who used conventional treatments had also used or were using an unorthodox treatment. Lerner and Kennedy (1992), in a national survey, found that 9% of cancer patients used alternative treatments. A Boston survey showed that 73% of patients with AIDS used alternative therapies in addition to prescription medications (Cohen et al. 1990).

Results can be tragic when alternative therapy prevents the use of conventional therapy. My first encounter with alternative medicine as an exercise in medical futility came when I was an intern at the Dartmouth-Hitchcock Medical Center in the late 1970s. A 13-year-old girl was admitted to the pediatrics ward for initial treatment for acute lymphocytic leukemia, a disease with an 85% rate of remission at that time. The parents were clearly distraught over the news of their daughter's cancer. The mother expressed her desire to have her daughter treated by a chiropractor, who claimed that he could cure the girl's cancer. Despite our pleas and arguments to the contrary, the mother took her daughter out of the hospital for spinal manipulation. The child was brought back several weeks later, when the mother reported that the chiropractor had told her that he could not do anything because the girl was not brought to him soon enough. My colleagues and I were appalled at the attempt to shift the guilt to the mother. Why had this mother reached out to an unconventional approach that provided no documented cure for leukemia? One can only suppose that she could not bear the possibility of letting go of her daughter and thus disregarded the measured prognosis given by the physicians and followed the advice of the chiropractor, who offered salvation.

Seriously ill patients are comparing the costs and quality of life offered by alternative therapy with the therapeutic benefits offered by conventional therapies. Their anxiety about death may cause them to reach out desperately for help and choose a promise of cure that may be offered by alternative therapists rather than the more scientific, measured estimate of chances of cure provided by physicians. Furthermore, patients may feel that conventional practitioners have not presented suitable options to them. Or they may prefer an unknown probability of benefit from unconventional therapy to the promise of limited benefit from conventional therapy.

Physicians also have feelings of helplessness that they must deal with.

Patients seeking emotional support may sense the scientific physician's pessimism and want to hear about treatments offered by optimistic, that is, alternative, practitioners.

Dr. Ann Moore, a breast cancer oncologist at the New York Hospital in New York City, surveyed the use of alternative therapies among patients with breast cancer in her clinic (personal communication). Of the 55 consecutive women who responded to her questionnaire

80% had switched to a low fat–high fiber diet

85% had started taking multivitamins, averaging four or five per day

25% took some form of "alternative medication," including shark cartilage, vitamin injections, Chinese herbs, immune protectors, homeopathic pellets, miatake mushrooms, and mistletoe injections

30% sought some form of alternative therapist, such as nutritionist, acupuncturist, psychotherapist, Gestalt therapist, Shiatsu masseuse, naturopath, Chinese herbalist, or consultation with Dr. Emanuel Revici, known for an alternative method

50% were using some form of alternative healing method, such as support groups (e.g., SHARE, ACS, Lesbian breast cancer group), visualization, imaging, positive thinking (e.g., the ideas of Dr. Bernie Segal, Norman Vincent Peale, or various inspirational tapes), yoga, crayon drawing, cold water swimming, prayer, or psychic healing.

Moore's informal survey puts a human face on statistics, reflecting human reactions to a disease such as breast cancer.

Should nutritional approaches be considered alternative medicine? If they promise a cure, yes. If they are offered as part of a regimen for prevention, no. Our understanding of the role of diet and vitamins has increased as we learn more about how they influence our health. Twenty years ago, nutritional approaches to disease were viewed as quackery, whereas today, they are gaining greater acceptance in conventional medicine.

Cassileth et al. (1984) reported that 75% of patients receiving alternative therapies informed their allopathic physician. Conventional physicians tended to disapprove of joint treatment approaches more frequently than did alternative practitioners. Patients reported that 4% of allopathic physicians refused to continue to care for patients who used both kinds of treatment, whereas none of the alternative practitioners refused to continue to treat the patient jointly. In contrast to Cassileth et al., Eisenberg et al. (1993) found that 72% of respondents who reported using alternative medical treatments did not inform their physicians.

There seems to be a difference of perception between patients and their conventional providers about the use of unproven cancer therapies (Lerner and Kennedy 1992). When physicians knew that their patient was using unconventional cancer treatments, 64% indicated that they discouraged their use. The final advice given to these patients was opposition by 52% of the physicians, acquiescence by 37%, and recommendation by 2%. This contrasted with the patients' perceptions. Of those patients who discussed the use of alternative treatments with their physician, 5% reported that their physician objected, 22% indicated that their physician acquiesced with the therapy, and 73% indicated that their physician recommended or approved of the alternative medicine. Clearly, many patients are choosing to use some form of alternative medicine even when their physicians disapprove, and many, sensing their physician's disapproval, do not tell the physician.

Evaluation of alternative therapies

Unlike new medications, alternative therapies are not subject to review by the Food and Drug Administration (FDA). Although most are probably harmless, colonic irrigation and coffee enemas have proved fatal, and high doses of vitamin B_6 have caused sensory neuropathy (Cassileth et al. 1991). A readily available Chinese herbal product injured the liver in some adults and may also be harmful to children (Delbanco 1994).

In an attempt to evaluate the effect of alternative treatments in patients with cancer, Cassileth et al. (1991) compared patients undergoing conventional cancer therapy at the University of Pennsylvania Medical Center with patients undergoing unproven cancer treatments at the Livingston-Wheeler Medical Clinic in San Diego, California. Patients were matched for age, sex, and type and stage of cancer. Patients undergoing unproven cancer therapy lived no longer than patients given conventional treatment and reported no enhanced quality of life during the course of disease.

Although members of the conventional medical community may not understand or approve of some aspects of alternative medicine, its use goes beyond prolongation of life. Patients are engaged in a healing process using approaches that we may not fully understand. Patients use alternative therapies for their potential benefit in controlling pain or other palliative effects and the perceived lack of side effects. Part of our job as physicians is to try to be supportive of our patients without compromising our principles when we agree to the use of alternative treatment. We must also deal with some of the unmet expectations of alternative medicine that anxious patients may have.

Certain sectors of the alternative medical community are anxious to achieve some level of acceptance by the conventional medical community. To succeed, the alternative medicine community needs to be precise in defining the questions that must be asked to assess the clinical efficacy of their proposed intervention. One of the myths that is promoted by some proponents of alternative medicine is that alternative medicine cannot be evaluated through conventional research methodologies. These methodologies are double-blind, randomized, placebo-controlled, multcentered clinical trials. Unfortunately, procedures such as meditation and acupunture cannot be evaluated in this way.

The National Cancer Institute (NCI) has developed a methodology for evaluating unconventional cancer therapies and poses important critical questions that must be addressed to convince the medical community and the public that this treatment has been fully explored. The required procedure is as follows: document the diagnosis of cancer, evaluate the appropriate anti-tumor or other clinical end point, do not provide other treatment for the disease, record previous anticancer treatments, document the sites of the patient's cancer, describe the patient's general medical condition, describe the treatment administered. A similar methodology has been developed by the National Institute for Allergy and Infectious Disease to evaluate unconventional AIDS therapies. Conventional medicine has been challenged in the same way by insurance companies and the managed care industry, who are asking that currently accepted treatments be proven effective. Managed care is predicated on the idea that doctors make imprecise decisions in determining clinical interventions and that their decision making can be normalized with formal guidelines. Managed care groups look to the medical literature on studies that challenge conventional medical wisdom. In the same way, consumers should look to reliable sources of medical information to help them make decisions affecting their care.

Patients' belief in the efficacy of treatment may itself be of great therapeutic benefit. This is particularly true of symptoms with a strong psychologic component, such as low back pain. Psychologic factors are even important in the progress of cancer. Spiegel et al. (1989) unexpectedly found that group therapy, in contrast to group education, lengthened the life of women with metastatic breast cancer.

Conclusion

We are in the midst of a tremendous change in the relationship between alternative (i.e., complementary) and orthodox medicine that is being forced by changes in patients' expectations and behavior toward conventional assumptions. This change can only be truly constructive if we explore the clinical evaluation of complementary medicine in a methodical, dispassionate manner, devoid of politics and bias, and if we then pass the information on to the health consumer. Since patients are using alternative cancer and AIDS treatments not only to aid the healing process but also as attempted cures, conventional medicine must try to understand alternative treatments as well as the reasons for their use.

The conventional physician may react to patients' discussions of alternative therapies or to their use with feelings of irritation and frustration. Such doctors perceive these treatments as futile at best – a waste of time, money, and hope – and as dangerous at worst – avoiding the best current scientific treatment and perhaps introducing toxins. They find it hard to stand by while their hard-earned knowledge and logic are challenged. This defensiveness, although understandable, is counterproductive. Technical expertise is no substitute for a warm supportive human interaction between the caregiver and the person in need. How effectively we as doctors deal with the spiritual dimension of patients' needs will directly influence how effective our biologic treatments will be. The challenge for doctors lies in rediscovering the art of listening; listening is a way of communicating caring. When we listen, we care, and when we do, the patient will benefit directly, and we will be better clinicians for it by becoming healers rather than curers.

References

Cassileth, B.R., Lusk, E.J., Guerry, D., et al. 1991. Survival and quality of life among patients receiving unproven as compared with conventional cancer therapy. *New England Journal of Medicine* 324:1180–5.

Cassileth, B.R., Lusk, E.J., Strouse, T.B., and Bodenheimer, B.J. 1984. Contemporary unorthodox treatments in cancer medicine: a study of patients, treatments and practitioners. *Annals of Internal Medicine* 101:105–12.

Cohen, C.J., Eisenberg, D.M., Mayer, K.H., and Delbanco, T.L. 1990. Prevalence of non-conventional medical treatments in HIV-infected patients: implications for primary care. *Clinical Research* 38:692A.

Delbanco, T.L. 1994. Bitter herbs: mainstream, magic and menace. *Annals of Internal Medicine* 121:803–4.

Eisenberg, D.M., Kessler, R.C., Foster, C., et al. 1993. Unconventional medicine in the United States. Prevalence, costs, and patterns of use. *New England Journal of Medicine* 328:246–52.

Lerner, I.J., and Kennedy, B.J. 1992. The prevalence of questionable methods of cancer treatment in the United States. *CA – A Cancer Journal for Clinicians* 42:181–91.

Spiegel, D., Bloom, J., Kraemer, H.C., and Gottheil, E. 1989. Effect of psychosocial treatment on survival of patients with metastatic breast cancer. *Lancet* 2: 888–91.

8

How culture and religion affect attitudes toward medical futility

MARY F. MORRISON, M.D., AND
SARAH GELBACH DEMICHELE, M.D.

Cultural and religious differences between the patient and the medical team are an underappreciated barrier to negotiating a sensitive and dignified process of dying for the patient. Medical professionals often have little understanding of their patients' views about health care decision making, life-sustaining technology, and the definitions of life and death (O'Rourke 1992). Impaired understanding because of cultural differences can make an already difficult struggle harder.

Cultures differ about definitions of life, death, and dying. For example, on the island of Vanatinai, southeast of Papua New Guinea, people are thought of as dead whom we would consider merely unconscious. Thus, it is possible for a person to die a number of times. On Vanatinai, considering someone to be dead generally leads to what we would consider medical neglect, but this disregard fits the cultural view (Rosenblatt 1993). In Hinduism, living is more than being alive, and quality of life plays an important part in the Hindu definition of life and death (Crawford 1995). Although brain death is a commonly accepted definition of death in the United States, Orthodox Jews do not accept it, and removing life support from a person who is brain dead is seen as tantamount to murder (Paris et al. 1995).

In times of crisis and when facing one's own mortality, religious and familial/cultural values are sources of strength and comfort. Recently, authors have disagreed about whether the Western emphasis on autonomy and full disclosure is respectful of dying patients with different cultural traditions. In the Asian, Hispanic, and other traditions, autonomy must be balanced against such values as family and community support and compassion. Full disclosure may be at variance with cultural beliefs about hope and wellness, and autonomous decision making may counter family-centered values (Gostin 1995). The patient's values determine whether it is beneficial or burdensome to be fully informed.

71

Furthermore, the caretakers' values and culture affect the interaction. Discussing, witnessing, and facilitating a dignified death are among the most difficult requirements of the medical profession. For physicians, nurses, and social workers to understand the motivations and beliefs driving a dying patient's thinking, they must understand their own beliefs, which is even more of a challenge.

Religious perspective on life, death, and initiation of life support

A central question for religions all over the world is what constitutes life. In the United States, these concerns have been evident in the public debate on abortion and withdrawal of life-sustaining technology. In addition to defining life, religion attempts to lift humans above pain, illness, and death (Henderson and Primeaux 1981) and help the believer to cope with grief and death. If all events are considered to be "God's will" or if the patient believes in an afterlife, he or she may accept adverse events and death with equanimity. However, some of the prominent medical–legal cases on end-of-life decisions reveal that religious family members may have great difficulty in withdrawing life support from a relative who is in a persistent vegetative state or who has a terminal illness.

Religious denominations that have addressed the issue of end-of-life decisions all affirm the sanctity of life. However, different religions have unique conceptions of the individual's obligation to accept treatment. Physicians are not commonly aware of the distinctions made by patients, their families, and their spiritual leaders.

Christianity

The belief in life after death is a firm belief of the Christian religion. "The Christian faith has its origin in what is considered a unique event in history. . . . The resurrection of Jesus as the Christ . . . is the central reality of the faith" (Mermann 1992). Although the body passes away, Christians believe that the soul will go on to another form of being, an eternal existence with God (Mermann 1992). Dying is filled with anxiety and dread. Death, however, represents a transformation and is less of a threat than it is in religions that do not believe in an afterlife.

In Catholicism, "ethically extraordinary" treatment does not have to be used simply to maintain life. However, treatment should not be initiated with the purpose of shortening life (Weir 1989). These principles are developed in the 1980 Roman Catholic Declaration on Euthanasia and The Catholic

Health Association Affirmation of Life (Grodin 1993). Declining further treatment in this situation reflects acceptance of the human condition and an unwillingness to use precious resources that are of little benefit. This view was extended to patients in the persistent vegetative states in the case of Karen Ann Quinlan, whose father was supported in court by his Catholic parish priest. The priest stated that the moral teaching of the Roman Catholic Church does not obligate one to resort to extraordinary means in cases of a persistent vegetative state in which the return to consciousness is virtually impossible.

Some Catholics believe that acceptance of suffering leads to spiritual growth, especially when one is nearing death. Suffering is thought to bring one closer to Christ, who was crucified in excruciating pain. They discourage the use of painkillers, which may cloud the consciousness of a terminally ill patient and thus diminish the patient's opportunity for spiritual progress and the expiation of guilt (Task Force on Pain Management, Catholic Health Association, 1993). Other Catholics believe that pain ought to be treated aggressively if that is a patient's wish, even if, as a by-product, a decrease in consciousness or respiratory function occurs (O'Rourke 1991; Task Force on Pain Management, Catholic Health Association 1993).

Protestant denominations also teach that a person may refuse life-sustaining measures that will only prolong the dying process. However, Protestant sects have different stances on active and passive euthanasia. To permit death with dignity, the Reformed Presbyterians, the American Baptist church of the USA, the Episcopal church, and Jehovah's Witnesses allow passive euthanasia by withdrawal of extraordinary means of life support when death is unavoidable, although they forbid active euthanasia. In contrast to most other Protestant denominations, Methodists believe that in certain situations, active euthanasia might be ethically permissible. Southern Baptists, the General Association of General Baptists, and the Lutheran church oppose all means of euthanasia. Christian Scientists believe in spiritual healing, so that euthanasia and the idea of medical futility are not a consideration (Crawford 1995: 94–7).

Judaism

This religion has a rigorous commitment to the sacredness of life. Since Orthodox Judaism strongly emphasizes the individual's obligation and responsibility to God, the concepts of self-determination and autonomy are irrelevant, and Orthodox Jewish patients must accept all treatment that will preserve every possible moment of life until the patient is ''very near'' death

(Kapp and Lo 1986). By Jewish law, the physician derives his authority directly from the Torah, and Orthodox physicians have a ''divine obligation'' to treat patients with all means available to preserve the sacredness of life (Crawford 1995:86–7).

Viewpoints on passive euthanasia vary. Some Orthodox Jewish theologians have a strong belief in hope and the possibility of recovering even from fatal diseases, whereas others permit the discontinuation of life support systems when death is impending and procedures or medications carry risks that outweigh their benefits.

Health care providers may be faced with patients and families who refuse to entertain the concepts of advance directives or do not resuscitate (DNR) orders, as their view is that life is sacred regardless of quality or burden (Kapp and Lo 1986). Facilitating the patient's access to family members and Jewish clergy members should be a priority. Since having a heartbeat is being alive, Orthodox Jews do not recognize brain death as death (Grodin 1993; Paris et al. 1995). However, brain death is recognized as death in the United States except in New Jersey, which by law permits religious exemption to brain death criteria.

Conservative and Reform Judaism support a more secular view of decision making and expand the idea of impending death to include conditions from which meaningful recovery is not probable. There is some support in the Torah for the view that the ''modern physician is not obligated to prolong the life of a terminal patient by artificial means, beyond food and water. As nature takes its course, the will of God is done'' (Crawford 1995). As in Orthodox Judaism, suicide and euthanasia are forbidden. There is concern about entering a ''slippery slope'' that leads to condoning suicide, euthanasia, and such horrors as the Holocaust (Kapp and Lo 1986).

Hinduism

Hindus oppose active euthanasia and consider it a form of suicide, which affects a Hindu's next life after reincarnation. By cutting short suffering, a person is purging his karma (destiny). He is fated to carry that same karma into the next life (Crawford 1995:109).

The Hindu tradition also supports pain control and active euthanasia, however. ''Concentration on religious thought at the moment of death'' apparently prevents suffering after death. Thus, for a ''good death,'' one must be ''in a psychologically balanced state of mind, composed and in control.'' Pain and suffering at the end of life can interfere with composure and perpetuate suffering into the next life (Crawford 1995:117–22). To understand the implications of medical futility in the Hindu tradition, it is important to recognize the Hindu view of the self–body relationship. The highest human value in Hinduism is spiritual enlightenment. When the physical base (the body) becomes detrimental to the spiritual path, the person has the religious right to determine the course of his earthly journey. The concept of reincarnation may modify the Hindu's perception of the tragedy of death, putting the focus on the quality of life not the inevitability of death (Crawford 1995).

Islam

In the Muslim tradition of many Middle Eastern countries, the family's definition of death needs to be considered. Thus, one Iranian family believed that because their brain-dead relative was warm and had a heartbeat, removing a ventilator would be murder. Families are expected to be demanding and to insist on a wide range of medical care to show concern for their loved one. Families of Muslim patients may want to shift the bed when removing life support so that the patient faces Mecca at death (Klessig 1992).

Buddhism

Like Hindus, Buddhists believe in reincarnation, and "in a sense, death becomes the highlight of life, a great opportunity for realizing pure enlightenment through attainment of the Buddha mind" (Irish, Lundquist, and Nelsen 1993:130). Buddhist teachings place a strong emphasis on a person's state of mind at the time of death because this influences their rebirth. There is a great need to be able to report that the patient was calm at the time of death. Family members may chant at the bedside or at a nearby temple with the intent of calming and protecting the dying. Buddhists in general do not advocate the use of medications, except in the case of extreme suffering and then only if the mind can remain clear (Irish et al. 1993:133).

Religious advance directives

The secular Western view of patient self-determination, autonomy, and control, especially in regard to medical decision making, can meet with significant opposition from patients of different religious backgrounds. This has led to the development of religious advance directives. The Halakhic Health Care Proxy allows patients to designate a decision maker who is knowledgeable about the teachings of the Halakha (Code of Jewish Law) if they themselves are unable to participate fully (Grodin 1993). The Jewish Health Care Proxy specifies that the patient wishes Orthodox law to be followed and, if necessary, that an Orthodox rabbi be consulted to assist in guiding decision making.

The Catholic Health Association Affirmation of Life has also developed an advance directive.

The use of special directives can be problematic, as their interpretation is subject to controversy and can be more restrictive than the patient intended. However, attempts to codify beliefs and religiously based intentions is valuable when the information is used as a foundation for further communication. Designating appropriate health care proxies and facilitating communication among patients, their agents, and health care providers is likely to serve the patient's wishes better (Grodin 1993).

Cultural and ethnic perspectives on life, death, and initiation and withdrawal of life support

Great comfort and strength can be derived from one's cultural background and traditions, especially during the process of dying. Cultural responses vary enormously, however. For example, although the usual reaction to loss is sadness, the Kaluli of Papua New Guinea express grief through anger and aggression (Rosenblatt 1993).

Although serious ethical issues can arise from contradictions between biomedical perspectives and the norms and values of different cultural groups (Muller and Desmond 1992), these ethical dilemmas have received little attention. Traditional medical training provides little or no education about the influence of culture on the practice of medicine or, in an even broader sense, about how discussions of end-of-life decisions should be conducted between a physician and a patient from a different culture. Language barriers also can cause great difficulty in end-of-life discussions and may mask hidden agendas that can sometimes be resolved by a professional translator.

Another clinical issue that is profoundly affected by culture is the perception and expression of pain in dying patients. Social research has shown that Italians tend to exhibit bodily symptoms readily and cope by dramatization. Irish cope by denial, and Scottish patients believe that they should bear discomfort as long as possible (Trill and Holland 1993). Physicians need to be tolerant of the cultural variations in expression of pain and desire for pain control and should avoid judgmental responses.

Alternative, nonbiomedical treatments may be important in coping with serious illness and dying in patients from some cultures. Examples of this include the use of acupuncture and Chinese medicine, traditional herbal medicine, and belief in spirits and certain rituals (see Chapter 7). No matter how acculturated the patient appears to be, at times of great stress, familiar systems that can help patients to cope need to be explored (Barker 1992). It is important for the physician to elicit information about health beliefs and non-Western health treatments to understand the psychosocial needs of the patient, the potential for noncompliance with the Western medical plan, and possible treatment interactions. Open and nonjudgmental inquiry is important in eliciting this information. The following sections explore specific cultural differences.

American

The United States is a religiously and culturally diverse nation. In 1992, the population distribution was 83% white, 12% African American, 3% Asian or Pacific Islanders, and 0.8% Native American or Eskimo. Immigrants were even more culturally diverse, with 37% of Asian origin (including Middle Eastern), 44% from Hispanic countries (South and Central America and Mexico), and 3% from Africa (US Bureau of the Census 1994:11, Table 8). With the ever changing ethnic mix in America, both patients and doctors may find themselves confused, baffled, and surprised by different customs and viewpoints. There is therefore no typical American view of life, death, and life support.

American Caucasian culture. The United States was founded on the principles of personal freedom of religion, speech, self-expression, and personal decision making, and, therefore, independence and self-sufficiency and open communication are emphasized. These tenets form the basis for the current support of open discussion and legislation about decisions made at the end of life and in situations of medical futility. Assisted suicide may, in this context, be seen as the ''pursuit of happiness.''

African American culture. Ethnicity and race appear to influence decision-making preferences and trust in the medical system at the end of life. Isolation has led many African Americans to reject some beliefs that are considered mainstream American values (Thomas 1981). Discrimination may be feared in hospital settings, increasing the wish to initiate or maintain life support in terminal illness. The strong family bonds that dominate the African American culture often are used as a protective measure against outside forces (Thomas 1981; Dula 1994).

Religion also provides ''hope, a place for belonging, a place for one to feel esteemed and a place for releasing pent-up emotions'' (Thomas 1981: 213). Forty-two percent of African Americans are Baptist (58% when including members of the National Baptist Conference), 25% are members of the Church of God and Christ, and 14% are African Methodist Episcopal (Horton and Smith 1990). The African American clergy are important sources of strength for sick and hospitalized patients.

Elderly African Americans tend to delay in seeking medical attention. Among the reasons are real and perceived barriers to treatment, over-representation in the lower socioeconomic brackets, less insurance coverage compared with others in their economic stratum, more serious chronic diseases, and more problematic lifestyles (Secundy 1994). African Americans who enter the primary care setting are three times more likely than Caucasians to desire more end-of-life care (Garrett et al. 1993; Caralis et al. 1993). This may result in part from more strongly held religious beliefs and faith in miracles, but there also appears to be a strong expectation of inadequate care because of race. Highly educated Caucasian patients were less likely than less well educated Caucasians to desire aggressive care at the end of life (Garrett et al. 1993); this was not true among African Americans, who wanted more end-of-life care at all educational levels. Communication and respect need to be actively cultivated by Caucasian physicians in end-of-life discussions with minority patients, since trust of physicians' decision making is an important issue.

Hispanic/Mexican/Latino cultures.   The extended family plays a large role in Hispanic culture, and families usually provide support by accompanying the patient to office and hospital visits. The concept of *personalismo* has been used to describe a person's unique significance within the context of the family network (Siefken 1993). This is ''a deep sense of being part of a network that comprises one's family as well as a sense of family as an extension of the person'' (Siefken 1993). The well-being of the family is thought to be more important than that of the individual. Doctors are often treated with unquestioning respect; to contradict a physician is considered rude, and patients may expect that doctors will make decisions (Klessig 1992).

Christian views are stressed – that death is determined by God's will and that suffering is an integral part of that process. In a study of Hispanics in the United States in primary care settings, 42% wanted their doctor to keep them alive regardless of how ill they were (Caralis et al. 1993). These numbers are similar to those for African Americans (37%) but much higher than those for non-Hispanic whites (14%), perhaps reflecting some distrust of the American medical establishment.

Mexican Americans did not want to be told about a terminal illness (Gonda and Ruark 1984; Blackhall et al. 1995) and were also less likely to feel bound to communicate this information to a loved one. Forty-five percent of an elderly Mexican American population believed that the family, not the patient, should be the primary decision maker in terminal care. Belief that the patient should be told the truth about the diagnosis correlated with the degree of acculturation (Blackhall et al. 1995).

Asian culture. The Asian concept of self is a familial self, as opposed to the individualized sense of self in Western cultures (Nilchaikovit et al. 1993). Boundaries between self and other are less rigidly drawn; one's life is interconnected with others, and there is a distinct sense of mutual obligation. The idealized physician–patient relationship in many Asian cultures is hierarchical, with the physician as an authority figure.

Communication style favors a more indirect approach, and there is more sensitivity to such means of communication within the family structure. This, combined with a strong respect for the educational/occupational hierarchy, may inhibit open communication with a physician. Death is believed to be a part of the normal life cycle, and within the family system, the ideal response is one of serenity, even to the point of denial (Nilchaikovit et al. 1993:46–47). A sense of ''closed awareness'' has been described, in which the medical staff and patient are aware of impending death, but discussions of this are avoided (Chang 1981). The family is intimately involved and is often present in medical settings – if necessary as interpreters but also as a filter to shelter the patient from a bad prognosis or diagnosis and the burden of decision making.

To engage in a discussion of prognosis or code status with a Chinese patient, as the ethics of American physicians dictates, is like casting a death curse, making the person despair and possibly die sooner. Disclosure to the patient of the specifics of the condition is thought to be a burden that is far outweighed by the benefit of continuing treatment. The insistence of American physicians on truth telling is perceived as dangerous and rude. When a patient's illness is life threatening, it is assumed that practitioners will talk with the family rather than with the patient, who is to be protected (Muller and Desmond 1992). Differing values of physicians and Asian family members can cause a breakdown of communication and mutual distrust.

Koreans, with Buddhist, Protestant, and Taoist influences, are generally opposed to stopping life support measures, as that is thought to be "interfering with God's will." In a study of elderly Americans of different ethnic backgrounds, Korean Americans were less likely than other Americans to believe that a patient should be told about a terminal prognosis and make decisions about life support. Instead, they believe that the family should make life support decisions (Blackhall et al. 1995). The strong sense of family loyalty requires parent's lives to be preserved by their children, and stopping life support may dishonor the family in the community even if it is the parent's wish. Thus, the children will be adamantly opposed to discontinuing life support even in futile situations (Klessig 1992).

Physicians in Japan, following long tradition, tend to be paternalistic, keeping patients ignorant of their condition and giving them little decision-making power (Feldman 1994). Patients mistrust physicians, although the norm of *enryo* dictates patient behavior in relationships: restraint, reserve, and lack of assertiveness in social interactions (Chang 1981). Therefore, traditional Japanese patients do not demand a strong voice in decision making.

There is no established policy on do not resuscitate (DNR) orders in Japan, and they may be used inappropriately. Thus, "futile CPR is often performed at the time of death in patients with terminal lung cancer" (Fukaura et al. 1995). Patients in Japan participated in the decision about DNR orders at a lower rate (5%) than in other countries (14%–41%), probably reflecting their paternalistic style of medicine. Physicians usually discussed end-of-life decisions with surrogates rather than with the patients themselves and performed CPR for the benefit of the surrogates (Fukaura et al. 1995).

Native American culture. There are approximately 350 different tribes in the United States. Identity is focused on the tribe or nation rather than on Native American ancestry in general. Values and beliefs vary greatly from nation to nation. For example, the Apache regard a dead person's body as an empty shell, whereas the Lakota speak to the body, visit it, and understand it to be sacred. Unlike most Native American nations, the Navajo do not believe in an afterlife (Brokenleg and Middleton 1993).

The Lakota find that death is often forecast by unusual spiritual or physical events. An accepted sign that a person will die soon is that she or he reports being visited in dreams by dead relatives. When a Lakotan dies, a substantial number of family and friends gather. Thus, when a young Lakota man was dying in the intensive care unit, 23 friends and relatives were at his bedside. This was perceived as being enormously supportive and respectful of their culture (Brokenleg and Middleton 1993).

In traditional Navajo culture, thought and language have the power to shape reality and control events. It is important to think and talk in a positive way, or "the Beauty Way." Discussion of negative information, such as issues of death and dying, is therefore potentially harmful. Nineteen of twenty-two Navajo said that advance care planning was a dangerous violation of traditional Navajo ways of thinking (Carrese and Rhodes 1995).

Gender

Few cultures share an egalitarian role for men and women; in most cultures, men are the primary decision makers for their female relatives (Henderson and Primaux 1981). In such male-centered cultures, women with serious or terminal illness may be concerned about their inability to perform household chores, and male family members may decide that it is not within their role to help with such chores or even with medical treatment given at home.

In the United States, there appear to be gender differences in court decisions about termination of life support. Miles and August (1990) report that in the absence of written directives, courts are more likely to construct patient preferences to terminate life support for men than for women. For female patients, helplessness and medical frailty summon aid, whereas for male counterparts, life-sustaining medical assistance is regarded as dehumanizing and likened to battery (Jecker 1994).

Courts were less likely to construct preferences on behalf of female patients because they treated prior evidence of women's values and choices as immature, emotional and uninformed, but considered men's choices and lifestyle decisions to be mature and rational, thus forming a more solid basis upon which to infer present preferences. (Jecker 1994)

It is thus likely that since a women's requests to forgo life-sustaining treatment are often discounted, other requests about end-of-life care may be minimized or ignored.

The role of physicians

In the United States, physicians are almost universally involved in the discussions of end-of-life decisions but often only when situations have reached a crisis point. These decisions would be much more effective if discussions were initiated early, allowing a more complete exploration of a patient's views of life, death, and life support and the optimal degree of involvement with family members. However, physicians themselves come from vastly different religions and cultures, with their own views and personality styles, and many other factors may impede this process as well.

Little is known about how the religious and cultural beliefs of the doctor affects a patient's decisions about terminal care. In an Australian study of the religious affiliation of physicians and their attitudes and practice of euthanasia, Baume et al. (1995:50) reported that

Of those identifying as agnostic or atheist who had been asked to hasten death, more than one third (34.6%) recorded that they had taken active steps to comply with such a request at least once, compared to just under a quarter (24.7%) of those who identified a religious affiliation. The ''non-theists'' were 1.6 times as likely to practice active voluntary euthanasia as were all ''theists''. Only 18 percent of those who identified themselves as Catholic, 28 per cent of Anglicans, 25 per cent of other Protestants, 22 per cent of other Christians, 35 percent of Jews and 35 percent of Moslems had taken active steps to hasten death.

Interestingly, in this study, a large percentage of medical practitioners identified themselves as agnostics or atheists. Assuming that the results can be extrapolated to physician attitudes in the United States, the religious practice of physicians is an important variable in terminal care. A physician who is uncomfortable with presenting all options for care because of religious beliefs is obliged to disclose that to the patient.

Conclusion

The following issues should be explored when a physician discusses terminal care preferences with patients from any culture or religion. What is the patient's religious and cultural background, and how important is that in end-of-life care? What are the patient's values and concerns about dying? What is the patient's definition of death? Who constitute the patient's support system, and in what way should they be involved in terminal care decisions? Who does the patient choose for making medical decisions when he is incompetent? The challenge to American physicians will be to understand and bridge the gulf between their own values on dying and those of their patients, whatever their beliefs. Although some differences may not be resolvable, patients and families deserve a meaningful and dignified process of death and dying.

References

Barker, J.C. 1992. Cultural diversity – changing the context of medical practice. *Western Journal of Medicine* 157:248–54.

Baume, P., O'Malley, E., and Bauman, A. 1995. Professed religious affiliation and the practice of euthanasia. *Journal of Medical Ethics.* 21:49–54.

Blackhall, L. J., Murphy, S. T., Frank, G., et al. 1995. Ethnicity and attitudes toward patient autonomy. *Journal of the American Medical Association* 274:820–5.

Brokenleg, M., and Middleton, D. 1993. Native Americans: adapting, yet retaining. In *Ethnic Variations in Dying, Death and Grief*, pp. 101–12. Washington, DC: Taylor & Francis.

Caralis, P., Davis, B., Wright, K., et al. 1993. The influence of ethnicity and race on attitudes toward advance directives, life-prolonging treatments and euthanasia. *Journal of Clinical Ethics* 4:155–65.

Carrese, J.A., and Rhodes, L.A. 1995. Western bioethics on the Navajo reservation. Benefit or harm? *Journal of the American Medical Association* 274:826–9.

Chang, B. 1981. Asian-American patient care. In *Transcultural Health Care*. Henderson, G., and Primeaux, M., eds., pp. 255–78. Menlo Park, CA: Addison Wesley.

Crawford, S.C. 1995. *Dilemmas of Life and Death. Hindu Ethics in a North American Context.* Albany, NY: State University of New York Press.

Dula, A. 1994. The life and death of Miss Mildred. An elderly black woman. *Clinical and Geriatric Medicine* 10:419–30.

Feldman, E. 1994. Culture, conflict and cost. *International Journal of Technology Assessment in Health Care* 10:447–63.

Fukaura, A., Tazawa, H., Nakajima, H., et al. 1995. Do-not-resuscitate orders at a teaching hospital in Japan. *New England Journal of Medicine* 333:805–8.

Garrett, J.M., Harris, R.P., Norburn, J.K., et al. 1993. Life-sustaining treatment during terminal illness: who wants what? *Journal of General Internal Medicine* 8: 361–8.

Gonda, T., and Ruark, J. 1984. *Dying Dignified. The Health Professional's Guide to Care.* Menlo Park, CA: Addison-Wesley.

Gostin, L.O. 1995. Informed consent, cultural sensitivity, and respect for persons. *Journal of the American Medical Association* 274:844–5.

Grodin, M.A. 1993. Religious advance directives: the convergence of law, religion, medicine and public health. *American Journal of Public Health* 83:899–903.

Henderson, G. and Primeaux, M. 1981. Religious beliefs and healing. In *Transcultural Health Care*. Henderson, G., and Primeaux, M., eds., pp. 185–195. Menlo Park, CA: Addison Wesley.

Horton, C.P., and Smith, J.C., eds. 1990. *Statistical Record of Black America*. Detroit, MI: Gale Research Inc.

Irish, D., Lundquist, K., and Nelsen, V.J., eds. 1993. *Ethnic Variation in Dying, Death, and Grief. Death Education, Aging and Health Care*. Washington, DC: Taylor & Francis.

Jecker, N.S. 1994. Physician-assisted death in the Netherlands and the United States: ethical and cultural aspects of health policy development. *Journal of the American Geriatrics Society* 42:672–8.

Kapp, M., and Lo, B. 1986. Legal perceptions and medical decision making. *Milbank Quarterly* 64 (Suppl. 2):163–202.

Klessig, J. 1992. Cross cultural medicine: a decade later. The effect of values and culture on life support decisions. *Western Journal of Medicine* 157:316–22.

Mermann, A.C. 1992. Spiritual aspects of death and dying. *Yale Journal of Biology and Medicine* 65:137–42.

Miles, S.H., and August, A. 1990. Courts, gender and ''the right to die.'' *Law, Medicine and Health Care* 18:85–95.

Muller, J.H., and Desmond, B. 1992. Ethical dilemmas in a cross-cultural context. A Chinese example. *Western Journal of Medicine* 157:323–7.

Nilchaikovit, T., Hill, J.M., and Holland, J.C. 1993. The effects of culture on illness behavior and medical care. Asian and American differences. *General Hospital Psychiatry* 15:41–50.

O'Rourke, K. 1991. Assisted suicide: an evaluation. *Journal of Pain and Symptom Management* 6:317–24.

O'Rourke, K. 1992. Pain relief: the perspective of Catholic tradition. *Journal of Pain and Symptom Management* 7:485–91.

Paris, J.J., Bell, A.J., and Murphy, J.J. 1995. Pediatric brain death: dead is dead. *Journal of Perinatology* 15:67–70.

Rosenblatt, P. 1993. Cross-cultural variation in the experience, expression, and understanding of grief. In *Ethnic Variations in Dying, Death, and Grief*, pp. 13–19. Washington, DC: Taylor & Francis.

Secundy, M.G. 1994. Lack of a moral consensus on health care: focus on minority elderly. In *The Ethics of Health Care for African Americans*, pp. 56–60. Westport, CT: Praeger.

Siefken, S. 1993. The Hispanic perspective on death and dying: a combination of respect, empathy and spirituality. *Pride Institute of Longterm Home Health Care* 12:26–8.

Task Force on Pain Management, Catholic Health Association. 1993. Pain management. Theological and ethical principles governing the use of pain relief for dying patients. *Health Progress* 74:30–9.

Thomas, D.N. 1981. Black American patient care. In *Transcultural Health Care*. Henderson, G., and Primeaux, M., eds., pp. 209–223. Menlo Park, CA: Addison Wesley.

Trill, M.D., and Holland, J. 1993. Cross cultural differences in the care of patients with cancer. A review. *General Hospital Psychiatry* 15:21–30.

U.S. Bureau of the Census. 1994. Statistical Abstract of the United States. Washington, DC: U.S. Government Printing Office.

Weir, R. 1989. *Abating Treatment with Critically Ill Patients*. New York, NY: Oxford University Press.

9

When religious beliefs and medical judgments conflict: civic polity and the social good

JOHN J. PARIS, S.J., PH.D., AND
MARK POORMAN, C.S.C., PH.D.

The futility debate

Medical futility as a justification for unilateral physician refusal of requested treatment is an enormous shift from the norm of shared patient–physician decision making (Alpers and Lo 1995). In the ordinary course of events, the joint decision process involves the physician making a diagnosis, forming a prognosis, and, on the basis of experience, providing a recommendation. The patient, using personal values, can accept or reject the proposed treatment. If the recommended treatment is rejected, the patient and physician might negotiate for another course of treatment. When agreement is not possible, the patient may go to another physician or – as one-third of Americans now do – seek help from nontraditional sources (Eisenberg et al. 1993).

The idea of shared decision making is itself a radical departure from the long-standing paternalist stance of medicine, which holds that the physician alone makes the medical choices. That standard was so well established in the early history of medicine that Hippocrates exhorted physicians to ''reveal nothing of the patient's future or present condition lest the patient falter and take a turn for the worse'' (Hippocratic Corpus 1923). Paternalism gradually gave way to patient involvement in medical decisions. Part of this process is the requirement that the patient give informed consent before any procedure can be undertaken. Under that standard, patients have a right to be informed about the range of available alternatives and to choose among those that are offered (Faden and Beauchamp 1986). Although the President's Commission (President's Commission 1983) reminds us that informed consent does not confer on patients the right to demand particular treatments, the emphasis on patients' rights and the extraordinarily high status given to autonomy over the last two decades have led to the belief among some physicians and bioethicists that autonomy involves not only the right of patients and their families to accept or decline a proposed therapy but also the right to whatever life-sustaining intervention they desire.

That belief finds support in both the medical and the bioethical literature. In a text on critical care, Raffin writes, "If family members or legal surrogates for the patient want every possible measure taken to keep the patient alive, professionals should comply with this request" (Raffin 1992:2185). In an editorial on the *Wanglie* case (*In re Helga Wanglie* 1991), Angell supports that position. Any other decision, she argues, would be callous, unwise, and "inimical to patient autonomy" (Angell 1991:511). She would condone other action only when, as in our earlier reported case of *Baby L* (Paris, Crone, and Reardon 1990), the decision appears to violate the best interests of a patient who left no guidance or who, as in the case of a child, was unable to do so. Wolf takes a similar position. For her, medical ethics demands "respect for patient autonomy even when the physician disagrees with the patient's decision" (Wolf 1992:280).

Veatch and Spicer take an even stronger stand. They hold that in cases involving life-sustaining treatment, the attending physician is obliged to provide the requested treatment if no physician can be found who is willing to do so. This holds true even if a surrogate's request "deviates intolerably" from established standards or is, from the physician's perspective, "grossly inappropriate" (Veatch and Spicer 1992:25). For them, any override of a surrogate's demands must come from "a socially legitimated authority commissioned to function as protection of incompetents in cases of extreme neglect or abuse." Veatch and Spicer would, in effect, require physicians "as a condition of the monopoly privileges of licensure" to follow whatever requests for life-prolonging treatments patients or families make as long as the measures are effective in extending life unless that request is countermanded by a court order.

With an approach in place that puts near total control in the hands of the patient, there is no moral legitimacy to a physician's refusal of requested treatment. The physician is reduced from moral agent – one with professional responsibilities and limits on what may legitimately be done – to an extension of the patient's (or family's) whims, fantasies, or unrealizable hopes and desires. Such a relationship not only distorts the physician's role as moral agent but might destroy the very autonomy that the emphasis on unlimited self-determination was designed to enhance.

That danger is compounded if a patient's or proxy's demands are couched in religious terms. In such instances, the physician's medical judgment is pitted against the most fundamental and basic values of the patient, values that generally preclude the collaborative process or integrity-preserving compromise favored as conflict resolution by several commentators (Splittig 1990; Nelson 1994; McCrary et al. 1994). Even Jecker and Schneiderman's thoughtful "ethic of care," with its emphasis on "stepping out of one's personal frame of reference into the other's" and on "sustaining the web of connection so that no one is left alone," fails against the ideologic thrust of fundamental beliefs (Jecker and Schneiderman 1995:155).

Jecker and Schneiderman concede that in the case of Helga Wanglie, where the husband's insistence on continued aggressive treatment was based on the belief that only God, not man, should take a life, it may not have been possible to alter the perceptions of family members. Part of the problem, as Schneiderman notes, is that in the past when patients or their families sought a miracle, they went to church and prayed to God, whereas today "they come to the hospital and demand it of the physician" (Schneiderman 1994:861). They want and expect, as it were, "salvation through science" and "immortality through medicine" (Midgley 1992). The difficulty with this apotheosis of medical goals is that it is impossible to subject them to challenge or negotiation.

Clash between religious values and medical judgment

Such a clash is seen in several of the major futility cases that have surfaced in the public arena. In *Wanglie*, for example, the husband, after stating that "physicians should not play God," rejected all attempts at negotiation concerning his wife's care. To him, the removal of life support would show lack of faith in God's ability to perform a miracle; it would be another sign of the moral decay in civilization (Miles 1991:513). Ms. Harrell, the mother of Baby K, took a similar position. As the trial transcript shows, she has a "firm Christian faith . . . [and] believes that God will work a miracle if that is his will. . . . God, and not other humans, should decide the moment of her death" (*In the matter of Baby K* 1993:1026). As she later put it in a television interview on NBC's Dateline, "The only way I would let Stephanie [Baby K] go is if I felt that is what God wanted" (Dateline 1995). That interview concluded with the mother reading from the Bible: "Plead my cause, oh Lord, with them that strive with me. Fight against them that fight against me."

In *Gilgunn v. Massachusetts General Hospital* (1995), the daughter of a 72-year-old comatose woman in five-system failure sued the physicians at the Massachusetts General Hospital for "emotional distress" caused by their failure to attempt cardiopulmonary resuscitation (CPR) on her mother. Her reasoning for demanding CPR despite the mother's multisystem failure was: "It is my religion that life is everything. Start the treatment and wait and see what is God's will" (*Gilgunn v. Massachusetts General Hospital* 1995:42).

A most dramatic clash between religious values and medical judgment occurs with some ultraradical religious believers who reject brain death criteria as a determination of death. Despite the fact that whole brain death is now uniformly recognized as the legal standard of death by statute or court decision in all 50 states and the District of Columbia (Goldberg 1988:1207, nn. 59–60), there are radical right to life supporters (Byrne, O'Reilly, and Quay 1979) as well as some ultra-Orthodox Jews (Rosner and Bleich 1979) who believe that "one whose heart still beats still lives; despite the irreversible cessation of brain function; and it would be an act of murder to disconnect such an individual from a respirator" (Zweibel 1989:49).

A clash between medical standards and ultraconservative Jewish beliefs about brain death occurred in a New York case involving a victim of a gunshot attack by an Arab militant against a vanload of rabbinic students from Rabbi Menachem Schneerson's ultra-Orthodox Lubavicher sect. One of the students, a 16-year-old boy, was declared brain dead shortly after admission to St. Vincent's Hospital. Rabbis for the boy's family told the physicians caring for him that their religion beliefs dictated that "he be kept on the support systems as long as his heart could beat on its own" (Paris, Bell, and Murphy 1995). Despite the fact that New York's highest court had adopted brain death criteria as the definition of death (*People v. Eulo* 1984), the physicians and administrators at the Catholic hospital were reluctant to exacerbate the politically dicey situation occasioned by an Arab attack on a Jewish group and so agreed to continue "life-support" on the brain-dead boy "within reason." The issue was rendered moot three days later when the boy's heart stopped.

The conflict between religious views and medical standards is not always so readily resolved. There are published reports in the literature of a 49-year-old New York man who "survived" 74 days of brain death before a court-ordered removal of his respirator (Parisi, Kim, and Collins 1982) and of a Florida girl whose brain-dead body was ventilated for some 13 weeks until cardiac failure ended the family's hope for a miracle (Paris et al. 1995). Even more dramatic is the report by Bernstein et al. (1989) of a 30-year-old, 15-week pregnant woman who was supported with intensive care for 107 days after diagnosis of brain death until at 32 weeks gestation she was delivered of a normal male infant by cesarean section.

Short of a theocracy in which the word of God embraces both sacred and secular law, the potential for clashes between religious beliefs and medical judgment is real and in need of resolution. What we have in these situations, as Callahan has observed, is a cultural "dilemma about the good society and whether such a society should leave crucial life and death decisions in the hands of individuals or let them be decided, at least in great part, by commonly shared, cultural notions of what is and is not" the appropriate medical response to a dying patient (Callahan 1994).

Role of patient autonomy

Since the *Cruzan* decision (*Cruzan v. Director* 1990), there is in the United States a social consensus that patients are free to decline any and all medical treatments. Still unresolved is the right of an individual to seek assistance in ending his own life (Paris 1992) and the pressing question of physician refusal of life-sustaining treatment (Paris et al. 1993). What is involved in the latter issue is not only the limits, if any, on the exercise of self-determination but also the role of professional integrity, the physician's commitment "to do no harm," and the more global question of the allocation of common resources.

Brody puts the first of these topics into context when he argues that in the setting of futility, the focus ought not to be control and power between patient and physician, but the social role of the physician as physician (Brody 1992: 176).

If patients felt that the only powers involved were charismatic and social, it might be fine to insist on the fully shared power to pick and choose the best therapy. But so long as patients accept that a part of the physician's power is Aesculapian, then they must accept that a practitioner within the Aesculapian craft is the only person qualified to say what is or is not an appropriate exercise of that craft. Someone who calls himself a physician, but who is constantly willing to compromise on valid modes of treatment in order to satisfy the wishes of a patient, is a fraud.

Without being able to exercise and assert judgment on the appropriateness of a requested treatment, the physician is transformed from one involved in a coherent practice with its own internal goals and defining rules into an individual who must exercise a technical skill whenever requested. This, as we noted in the report on Baby L, could result in physicians being forced by surrogates to impose painful interventions on incompetent patients without affecting the patient's underlying condition (Paris 1990). Such brutalizing and inhumane action would in the hands of anyone but a physician be labeled torture; it is, we believe, abuse no matter the source. As such it violates the

first and most fundamental precept of the physician: primum non nocere –
first do no harm (Hippocratic Oath 1986).

The unrestricted claims of an individual to common resources raises issues
that by their very nature transform the conflict between religious views and
medical judgment from a clash between individual patient and physician values into a matter of public concern. It is no longer merely a question of
competing patient versus professional norms but a public assessment of the
relation of an individual's goals to the common good.

Individual preferences versus common good

The tension between individual rights or preferences and the pursuit of the
common good is addressed throughout the history of Western philosophical
and theological ethics. For Plato, the *polis* is founded for the good of the
whole and not for the exceptional welfare of any one group (Plato). Aristotle
reserves the term "just" for "those things which produce and preserve the
happiness of the social and political community" (Aristotle), and Thomas
Aquinas later reiterates that notion, emphasizing that as every imperfect part
is ordered to the perfect whole, law properly addresses the universal happiness of the whole community as the perfect expression of concern for the
individual person (Aquinas). St. Augustine's "commonwealth" is only
achieved when justice is construed as consent to law based on a "common
sense of right" (Augustine).

The common good is also found in specifically religious precepts. In their
synopsis of Catholic social teaching, Henriot, DeBerri, and Schultheis identify the common good as one of the "major lessons" of the tradition and
define it as the "sum total of all those conditions of living – economic,
political, cultural – which make it possible for women and men readily and
fully to achieve the perfection of their humanity," noting that "[i]ndividual
rights are always experienced within the context of the promotion of the
common good" (Henriot et al. 1988). Pope John XXIII's exhortation in the
encyclical *Pacem in Terris* exemplifies this (John XXIII 1963:213).

Individual citizens and intermediate groups are obliged to make their specific contributions to the common welfare. One of the chief consequences of this is that they
must bring their own interests into harmony with the needs of the community, and
must dispose of their goods and services as civil authorities have prescribed, in accord
with the norms of justice, in due process and within the limits of their competence.

Given this established ethical tradition, we turn our attention to the relationship of the common good to religious practices of individual persons.

Some insight into the resolution of that issue has been provided by the United States Supreme Court's rulings on what, if any, restrictions may be imposed on religious practice. In one of its earliest rulings on freedom of religion, the Supreme Court, in the process of upholding a ban in the territory of Utah against the Mormon practice of polygamy – a practice mandated by that sect's edicts "under pain of eternal damnation" – ruled that there is and must be a distinction between one's beliefs, which are to be untrampled in our Constitutional scheme of things, and public practices, which of necessity must be regulated to protect the common welfare. As the Court put it in its 1879 opinion in *Reynolds v. United States*: "Congress was deprived of all legislative power over mere opinion, but was left free to reach actions which were in violation of social duties or subversive of good order" (*Reynolds v. United States* 1879:151).

The distinction that protected beliefs but allowed regulation of public actions was reiterated in a 1940 Jehovah's Witness case, *Cantwell v. Connecticut*, when the Court, in words still frequently cited, ruled that the First Amendment clause on Freedom of Religion "embraces two concepts – freedom to believe and freedom to act." "The first," it declared, "is absolute, but in the nature of things, the second cannot be" (*Cantwell v. Connecticut* 1940:298). The only restriction on the state's power to regulate religious practices to protect public safety and well-being is the requirement that the regulations be neutral in their application (*Church of Lukumi* 1993). That is, they cannot be designed to discriminate against a particular religious practice.

The well-established policy in the United States that an individual does not have an absolute right to practice his or her religion free from all government interference or constraint finds support from both secular and religious commentators on the role of religion in civil society (Hollenbach 1993). Rawls, the eminent philosopher of liberal society, describing the religious and philosophical pluralism of modern democratic societies, notes that the multiplicity of beliefs "is not a mere historical condition that will soon pass away" (Rawls 1987). Consequently, he observes, there is no possibility of agreement or consensus on what constitutes the "good life," short, of course, of a totalitarian imposition of the views of one group or another. In a secular democratic state, the way to deal with religious diversity and deeply held religious differences on the meaning of life, Rawls believes, is what he labels "the methods of avoidance" (Rawls 1987:12). This requires that, in the political life, "we try, so far as we can, neither to assert nor to deny any religious, philosophical or moral views, or their associated philosophical accounts of truth and the status of values." In sentiments that echo those of the Supreme Court's *Cantwell* opinion, Rawls maintains that although every individual must be free to hold his or her own view of the good life, those views are and of political necessity must be confined to personal conviction; they cannot be the basis of public policy. Rorty concurs in the argument that such convictions must "be reserved for private life" (Rorty 1988).

Hollenbach, a leading Catholic commentator on the role of communitarian and social values, quotes John Courtney Murray to the effect that "Whether we like it or not, we are living in a religiously pluralist society at a time of spiritual crisis; and the alternatives are the discovery of social unity, or destruction" (Hollenbach 1989:78). Hollenbach believes that without social unity, without some agreed-on social consensus on a vision of the human good, we cannot survive as a community. One threat to that consensus would be religion conceived of as a rigid set of beliefs held on nonrational grounds. From such a perspective, Hollenbach observes, "religion is very likely to be a source of division [and] conflict" and, as such, is "inherently uncivil" (Hollenbach 1993:894).

For Hollenbach, a consensus on the larger meaning of deeply held issues of fundamental importance demands that the believer must enter into dialogue with the broader civil society and be prepared to listen and, if necessary, to modify and even change his or her position. That is, religious beliefs and policy conclusions are not and, in the scheme of things in a pluralistic democracy, cannot be immediate and direct correlates. Thus, for him, social policy requires not merely a tolerance of religious beliefs or a laissez faire attitude toward them but a serious and sustained engagement of religious views and the more general civic order. Hence, a "closed communitarian" stance by which one's religious traditions and claims are intelligible only to other church members and not to the wider community's representatives can make but a minimal contribution to the common good (Hollenbach 1995).

A contrast to a "closed communitarian" stance is the position found in the introductory chapter of "Economic Justice for All," the U.S. Catholic bishops' pastoral letter on the economy (National Conference 1986). The bishops describe a dual intent for their project.

. . . to provide guidance for members of our own Church as they seek to form their consciences. . . . At the same time, we want to add our voice to the public debate. . . . We seek the cooperation and support of those who do not share our faith or tradition. The common bond of humanity that links all persons is the source of our belief that the country can attain a renewed public moral vision.

Even as they hope to teach and influence other believers through the distinctive claims of their own religious tradition, the bishops are nonetheless engaged by the more inclusive prospect that "the common bond of humanity that links all persons'' will be the foundation for a public moral vision. In such an engagement, as Tracy puts it, the believer's ''convictions must be brought into mutually critical correlation with understandings based on human experience and reasoned reflection on this experience'' (Tracy 1994).

Application to futility cases

This theologic perspective is not shared by all believers. Mrs. Wanglie's husband would have no truck with the moral decay of compromise. Baby K's mother did not enter into ''mutual critical'' assessment of her position with the physicians treating her daughter. To her, they were ''enemies'' to be fought, not advocates of a competing but acceptable view of life. Much like the ultraconservative Jews who reject the notion of brain death, for Baby K's mother, equating the ''life'' of her anencephalic daughter to ''death'' is blasphemy. In her eyes, all life, regardless of its compromised quality, is equally precious in the divine plan. Any compromise on that issue is excluded as a betrayal of God's command.

The difficulty presented by such religious views is that in the cases cited, the physicians' position is equally a matter of commitment and integrity. It was not physician intransigence or financial concern – in each of these cases there was full payment for the requested treatment – but a moral stand on what the good physician is and does that led the physicians in *Baby L* (Paris et al. 1990), *Baby K*, and *Wanglie* to say ''no.'' In the latter two cases, as well as in the case involving extracorporeal membrane oxygenation we have described elsewhere (Paris et al. 1993), no other physician could be located who was willing to treat the patient as the proxy demanded.

In such an impasse, Veatch and Spicer argue that ''it is a legitimate compromise to impose [on the physician] a limited duty to treat with life-prolonging technology as a condition of the monopoly privileges of licensure'' (Veatch and Spicer 1992:28). In a subsequent essay, Veatch modifies that ''social contract'' argument to read, ''If society is giving medical professionals exclusive monopoly privileges in conjunction with licensure, *it would be wise* for them to extract certain promises at the time the privileges are given'' [emphasis added] (Veatch 1994:873).

In an argument that implies that it is physicians' class and social bias that is producing the conflict with religious conscience, Veatch and Spicer argue that they will hold physicians to a ''legitimate'' compromise of their professional values ''[o]nly in a period, while we strive to better coordinate the values of professionals and patients'' (Veatch and Spicer 1992:28). At a time when we have an adequate number of physicians who, for example, share the proposition that if requested, physicians should provide aggressive treatment for an anencephalic infant, there would be no need to compel the unwilling physician to do so.

Veatch and Spicer's argument devalues the professional integrity and conscience of the individual practitioner. This is no surprise in Veatch (1994), who holds that medicine has no internal morality. Those who view medicine as a higher calling – one that in the words of the Hippocratic Oath requires the physician to act always for the benefit of the patient according to "my skill and my judgment" – find that conscience, as well as the technical skill of the physician, is a factor in the social equation.

The moral conscience of the physician as medical practitioner has been recognized by both courts and legislatures. The leading judicial precedent is the landmark opinion in *Brophy v. New England Sinai Hospital*, in which the Massachusetts Supreme Judicial Court, in an opinion that upheld the right of an unconscious Paul Brophy to be free of unwanted life-sustaining medical treatment, ruled that individual physicians could not be required to remove or clamp Brophy's feeding tube "contrary to their view of their ethical duty toward their patient" (*Brophy v. New England Sinai Hospital* 1986:441). In the course of its opinion, the Supreme Judicial Court also ruled that a hospital and its staff "should not be compelled . . . [to act] contrary to [their] moral and ethical principles, when such principles are recognized and accepted within a significant segment of the medical profession and the hospital community."

The Virginia Health Care Decisions Act also provides support for physicians' rejection of patient or family demands for medical treatment (*Va. Code Ann.* 1992:Art 541-2990).

Nothing in this article shall be construed to require a physician to prescribe or render medical treatment to a patient that the physician determines to be medically or ethically inappropriate. However, in such a case, if the physician's determination is contrary to the terms of an advance directive of a qualified patient or the treatment decision of a person designated to make the decision under this article, the physician shall make a reasonable effort to transfer the patient to another physician.

Conclusion

The widely divergent cross-cultural differences and varying religious views in a pluralistic democratic society require that physicians approach the issue of treatment decisions with openness and sensitivity. In encounters with the patient, the physician should listen to, adapt, and, if possible, adopt the patient's perspective. As many of the cases that have emerged in the futility debate demonstrate, however, individual religious perspectives may not only challenge but conflict – sometime violently – with medical standards and the prevailing view of the social good.

When such conflict occurs, and the most sensitive attempts at an "ethic of care" fail to resolve the clash of private views and public values – those not of the individual practitioner but of the profession as a whole – the distinction between religious beliefs and actions found in the Supreme Court's opinion in *Reynolds* provides helpful guidance. The legislature is and must be able to regulate and control "actions which [are] in violation of social duties or subversive of good order" (*Reynolds v. United States* 1879: 152).

References

Alpers, A., and Lo, B. 1995. When is CPR futile? *Journal of the American Medical Association* 273:156–8.

Angell, M. 1991. The case of Helga Wanglie – a new kind of "right to die" case. *New England Journal of Medicine* 325:511–12.

Aquinas, T. 1254–56. On the essence of law. *Summa Theologica* II-I, Question 90, Article 2.

Aristotle. 1962. *Nicomachean Ethics*, Book V:1129 (trans. by Ostwald, M.), p. 113. Indianapolis: Bobbs-Merrill.

Augustine. 1986. *City of God*, Book XIX, Chap. 21 (trans. by Bettenson, H.), p. 883. New York: Penguin Books.

Bernstein, I.M., Watson, M., Simmons, G.M., et al. 1989. Maternal brain death and prolonged fetal survival. *Obstetrics and Gynecology* 74:434–7.

Brody, H. 1992. *The Healer's Power*. New Haven: Yale University Press.

Byrne, P.A., O'Reilly, S., and Quay, P.M. 1979. Brain death: an opposing viewpoint. *Journal of the American Medical Association* 242:1985–90.

Callahan, D. 1994. Necessity, futility, and the good society. *Journal of the American Geriatrics Society* 42:866–7.

Dateline NBC, March 14, 1995. Interview with Ms. Katrina Harrell, Transcript 1995 WL 6295785 (1995).

Eisenberg, D.M., Kessler, R.C., Foster C., et al. 1993. Unconventional medicine in the United States: prevalence, costs, and patterns of use. *New England Journal of Medicine* 328:246–52.

Faden, R., and Beauchamp, T.L. 1986. *A History and Theory of Informed Consent*. New York: Oxford University Press.

Goldberg, C.K. 1988. Choosing life after death: respecting religious beliefs and moral correction in near death decisions. *Syracuse Law Review* 39:1197–260.

Henriot, P.J., DeBerri, E.P., and Schultheis, M.J. 1988. Catholic social teaching: our best kept secret. Maryknoll, NY: Orbis, 20–21.

Hippocratic Corpus (1923). 1977. In *Ethics in Medicine*. Reiser, S.J., Dyck, A.J., and Curran, W.J. eds. Cambridge: MIT Press.

Hippocratic Oath. 1986. In *Biomedical Ethics*, 2nd ed. Mappes, T.A., and Zembaty, J.S., eds. New York: McGraw-Hill, vol. 54.

Hollenbach, D. 1989. The common good revisited. *Theological Studies* 50:70–94.

Hollenbach, D. 1993. Contexts in the political role of religion: civil society and culture. *San Diego Law Review* 309: 887–901.

Hollenbach, D. 1995. The common good in the postmodern epoch: what role for theology? Paper presented at the Annual Convention of the College Theology Society, Worcester, Massachusetts, June 1, pp. 17–18.

Jecker, N.S., and Schneiderman, L.J. 1995. When families request that "everything possible" be done. *Journal of Medicine and Philosophy* 20:145–63.

John XXIII. *Pacem in Terris*. (April 11, 1963). 1976. In *The Gospel of Peace and Justice*. Gremillion, J., ed., p. 213, paragraph 53. Maryknoll, NY: Orbis.

McCrary, S.V., Swanson, J.W., Youngner, S.J., et al. 1994. Physicians' quantitative assessments of medical futility. *Journal of Clinical Ethics* 5:100–5.

Midgley, M. 1992. *Science as Salvation: A Modern Myth and Its Meaning*. New York: Routledge.

Miles, S.H. 1991. Informed demand for "non-beneficial" medical treatment. *New England Journal of Medicine* 325:512–15.

National Conference of Catholic Bishops. 1986. Economic justice for all: pastoral letter on Catholic social teaching and the U.S. economy, pp. 13–14. Washington, DC: NCCB.

Nelson, J.L. 1994. Families and futility. *Journal of the American Geriatrics Society* 42:879–82.

Paris, J.J. 1992. Active euthanasia. *Theological Studies* 53:113–26.

Paris, J.J., Bell, A.J., and Murphy, J.J. 1995. Pediatric brain death: dead is dead. *Journal of Perinatology* 15:67–70.

Paris, J.J., Crone, R.K., and Reardon, F. 1990. Physicians' refusal of requested treatment: the case of Baby L. *New England Journal of Medicine* 322:1012–14.

Paris, J.J., Schreiber, M.D., Statter, M., et al. 1993. Beyond autonomy: physicians' refusal to use life-prolonging extracorporeal membrane oxygenation. *New England Journal of Medicine* 329:354–7.

Parisi, J.E., Kim, R.C., Collins, G.H., and Hilfinger, M.F. 1982. Brain death with prolonged somatic survival. *New England Journal of Medicine* 306:14–16.

Plato. 1968. *The Republic*. Book IV:420b (trans. by Bloom, A.), p. 98. New York: Basic Books.

President's Commission for the Study of Ethical Problems in Medicine and Biomedical and Behavioral Research. 1983. *Deciding to Forego Life-Sustaining Treatment: Ethical, Medical, and Legal Issues in Treatment Decisions*. Washington, DC: Government Printing Office.

Raffin, TA. 1992. Perspectives on clinical medical ethics. In *Principles of Critical Care*. Hall, J. B., Schmidt, G.A., and Wood, L.D.H., eds. pp. 2185–204. New York: McGraw-Hill.

Rawls, J. 1987. The idea of overlapping consensus. *Oxford Journal Legal Studies* 7: 1–18.

Rorty, R. 1988. The priority of democracy to philosophy. In *The Virginia Statute for Religious Freedom: Its Evaluation and Consequences in American History*. Peterson, M.D., and Vaughn, R., eds. pp. 257–63. New York: Cambridge University Press.

Rosner, F., and Bleich, J.D. 1979. *Jewish Bioethics* New York, Hebrew Publishing.

Schneiderman, L.J. 1994. The futility debate: effect versus beneficial intervention. *Journal of the American Geriatrics Association* 42:853–86.

Splittig, B.M. 1990. The difference: compromise and integrity in ethics and politics. Lawrence, KS: University of Kansas Press.

Tracy, D. 1994. Catholic classics in American liberal culture. In *Catholicism and Liberalism: Contributions to American Public Philosophy*. Douglas, R.B., and Hollenbach, D., eds. pp. 196–213. New York: Cambridge University Press.

Veatch, R.M. 1994. Why physicians cannot determine if care is futile. *Journal of the American Geriatrics Society* 42:871–4.

Veatch, R.M., and Spicer, C.M. 1992. Medically futile care: the role of the physician in setting limits. *American Journal of Law & Medicine* 18:15–36.

Wolf, S.M. 1992. Toward a theory of process. *Law, Medicine & Health Care* 20: 278–89.

Zweibel, D. 1989. Accommodating religious objections to brain death: legal considerations. *Journal of Halacha and Contemporary Society* 17:49–68.

Cases and statutes

In the Matter of Baby K, 832 F. Supp. 1022 (E.D. Va. 1993).

Brophy v. New England Sinai Hospital, 398 Mass., 417, 497 N.E. 2d 626 (1986).

Cantwell v. Connecticut, 310 U.S. 296 (1940).

Church of Lukumi Babalu Aye, Inc., 113 S. Ct. 2217 (1993).

Cruzan v. Director Missouri Department of Health, 110 S.Ct. 2841 (1990).

Gilgunn v. Massachusetts General Hospital, Suffolk County Superior Court, 42 (1995).

People v. Eulo, 63 NY 2d 341, 472 N.E. 2d 298 (1984).

Reynolds v. United States, 98 U.S. 145 (1879).

In re Helga Wanglie: Fourth Judicial District (Dist. Ct., Probate Ct., Div.) PX-91–283. Minn., Hennepin County (1991).

Va. Code Ann. Ch. 29 Art. 541–2990 (1992).

10

Conflict resolution: experience of consultation-liaison psychiatrists

JAMES J. STRAIN, M.D., STEPHEN L. SNYDER, M.D., AND MARTIN DROOKER, M.D.

Medical futility often stimulates intense conflicts among medical/surgical patients, their families or surrogates, health care staff, medical–legal–financial systems, and ethical standards, including the allocation of scarce resources. These conflicts may be particularly intense when the patient is uncooperative or provocative (Groves 1979). Consultation-liaison (C/L) psychiatrists frequently are asked to help resolve such conflicts. The C/L psychiatrist is a member of the medical/surgical team who works directly with the patient and his doctor (i.e., consultation) and also influences the team's decisions through interactions with the rest of the patient's caretakers (i.e., liaison).

Specifically, the C/L psychiatrist (Strain and Grossman 1975):

1. Identifies patients at risk of or evidencing psychiatric or psychosocial difficulty
2. Treats patients in conjunction with the medical/surgical/nursing team
3. Suggests appropriate follow-up and aftercare of psychiatric problems
4. Addresses staff conflict(s) over patient care

Because of their background and experience in understanding human behavior, C/L psychiatrists are accustomed to dealing with conflicts relating to medical futility. Although each medical situation is unique, situations of futility have in common that the individuals involved have been deprived of a basic emotional tool, that of taking action. Being able to act effectively in the world provides a person with an outlet for aggression and is associated with feelings of confidence, self-esteem, independence, and safety. When effective action is impossible, as in a situation of medical futility, the individual may feel frustrated, angry, and vulnerable. Conflicts involving aggression frequently surface strongly. The C/L psychiatrist often can assist by helping the individual to tolerate inactivity or by shifting the focus from physical to psychologic activity, such as mourning or working through.

98

Dilemmas of patients and families

At times, it is the family who demands medical procedures, despite the efforts of doctors to convince them that all such efforts are in vain.

An 82-year-old patient

An 82-year-old man with prostate cancer, lung cancer, severe emphysema, and increasingly debilitating dementia was admitted to the emergency room with rapid heart and respiratory rates, falling blood pressure, and a decreasing level of awareness. The patient's condition was stabilized after two hours. Two weeks earlier, when widespread liver metastases were discovered, the family had been asked if they wished to sign a do not resuscitate (DNR) order. The son had thought that he could not let his father go and that the hospital staff should do everything they could to keep him alive, even just a few more days and even if the father had limited mental capacity. In the emergency room, the family again refused to authorize a DNR despite the patient's deteriorating condition.

The next day, as the blood pressure fell from 70/50 to 50/30, the C/L psychiatrist suggested that the patient's physician ask the family once more to sign a DNR order, tell them that treatment would be futile, and warn them that if a full code was called, the father's ribs might be fractured, and he would be pushed, pulled, and defibrillated to no avail. At the last moment, the son finally agreed that there was no point in continuing if that was what was going to happen. Only at this last request, with the father's condition painfully apparent and a frank confrontation of what resuscitation meant, was the son able to forgo futile procedures and let his father die.

The C/L psychiatrist was aware that the family, particularly the son, was not able to assimilate the reality of the father's condition. The psychiatrist was also aware, however, that the family had not been confronted with a full description of what the father would go through. He thought that the son might finally be reached by a clear statement that cardiopulmonary resuscitation (CPR) would only forestall death briefly and would unnecessarily traumatize the father's body. It was necessary to go this far to prevent medically futile activity.

For this son, loving his father meant taking every possible action to help him. Not taking action meant abandoning or hurting the father. It was only when the son understood that resuscitating his father would also mean hurting him that he was able to face the inevitability of his father's death. Futile situations commonly stimulate intense guilt in family members, who may go to great lengths to avoid actions that make them feel guilty.

A similar situation had a less opportune outcome for another, much younger patient.

An AIDS patient

Mr. A. had AIDS and was near death from widespread Kaposi's sarcoma. The family and patient were adamant that they would not sign a DNR because he was a young man of only 25. As in the preceding case, both patient and family wanted to preserve every moment of life that they could. In addition, the patient was convinced that he could improve and that signing a DNR would cause his premature death. As his condition worsened and death appeared imminent, another request not to pursue CPR was refused. When the patient's heart arrested an hour later, it was necessary for the staff to go through the entire resuscitation procedure, even though they knew that this effort was futile and that they were being unnecessarily exposed to contaminated blood.

In this situation, the wish for even one minute of life was so pervasive that confronting the patient and the family with the exigencies of his medical situation did not change their feelings or their belief that he might recover. The patient could not sign for his own death, as he could not accept what was going to happen. The wish to live, the belief in the fantasy of making it despite the claims of the doctors, was too powerful to be affected by the confrontation with reality. At the same time, the physicians were reluctant to say to the patient, ''Don't you know that you are dying, and all of these efforts are to no avail?''

In the case of Mr. A., the physicians saw an even more negative side to the futile procedure: they would be exposed to a risk that could prematurely terminate their own lives. They were angry that the patient's lack of reason not only put him and themselves through an unnecessary exercise but also placed them in danger. How could a patient be so ungrateful and subject them to harm when no good for him would come from their efforts?

The medical staff is understandably unhappy to comply when the patient and family demand tests that will offer neither benefit nor useful knowledge. These demands often arise from patients' and families' misunderstanding, fears that something has been overlooked, obsessional need to check over and over again, or a lack of faith and trust in the medical caregiver. Families may use all possible means to avoid guilt over abandoning the patient.

Often patients may be unwilling to shift from a futile approach to a more fruitful one.

A woman with abdominal pain

Mrs. T., a 32-year-old married mother of two, had had abdominal pain for six years, with repeated examinations and hospitalizations and repeated normal abdominal and pelvic CT scans. The pain had begun when she was delivered of an unwanted child. She had always believed that the delivery should have been by cesarean section, as the labor was so prolonged and difficult. During the present admission for abdominal pain, physicians had ordered another CT scan, which was negative. The patient insisted that the doctors do yet another scan, as they might have missed something. She thought that the doctors were not taking adequate care of her and that she could not go on with this discomfort.

The psychiatrist attempted to show the patient that her pain might be intensified by other causes, including her feelings of anger at having had a second child so soon and undergoing a prolonged and painful delivery, and that her symptoms – disturbances in eating, sleeping, libido, and energy – could be due to a depression. Despite this, she insisted on yet another CT scan and threatened to leave the hospital for another medical center if it were denied. Like many patients with depression, she was convinced that she had a physical ailment that the doctors had not yet detected. The pain was so ''real'' that it could not be ''in her head.''

Patients' demands for tests that would be futile in assisting assessment and diagnosis or developing a treatment plan can threaten the doctor–patient relationship. Offering another explanation for the symptom(s) may encourage the patient to accept an alternative approach. Often, however, the patient may defeat the physician who attempts to offer such help, as in this case.

Caregivers' dilemmas

The psychiatrist can be of great help to physicians and staff in recognizing and dealing with behaviors that are not in the best interest of the patient or themselves (Strain and Grossman 1975). Spikes and Holland (1975) have described three dysfunctional reactions of caregivers when they confront dying patients and their families.

Overtreatment

The physician may overtreat the patient, order one more test, pursue another operative procedure or invasive examination, or try yet another chemotherapeutic regimen in an overzealous need to do something for the patient. Not only does this put more stress on the patient, at times creating more pain and suffering, but also the overtreatment is often a treatment for the physician and not the patient.

A colleague as patient

The house staff were working in a constant rotation to care for an intern in their group. He became ill with infectious hepatitis following a needlestick after drawing blood from a patient and now lay comatose in their intensive care unit (ICU). His closest peers were in constant attendance, as was his new wife. On the seventh hospital day, his blood tests showed widespread destruction of the liver. On the eighth day, his electroencephalogram (EEG) was flat, and the young doctor had to be maintained on a ventilator. Two days later, the house staff refused to shut off the life support although his body was decomposing and his wife found it almost impossible to visit her husband. Finally, a world expert in liver disease who was visiting the hospital came to the ICU and informed the young staff doctors that she had never seen a patient with a flat EEG recover; in essence, their beloved colleague was brain dead. The only appropriate medical course was to shut off the machines and let him go. At last, the young doctors agreed and said goodbye to their colleague and friend. It was futile to go on.

The C/L psychiatrist had worked with the physicians and the ICU staff and was careful not to interfere with the house staff's wish to do everything they could for their friend – not to give up on him, as they would not want their colleagues to give up on them. In fact, to allow the house staff to work through this tragedy, the attending physicians did not take over the case, giving the demoralized staff as long as they needed to make the decision. Without the medical expert's intervention, the house staff might not have been able to stop when they finally did. It was only by identifying with a much respected older colleague that these young physicians could finally bear their helplessness in the face of death and begin to mourn the loss of their friend. The medical care during the last five days of this young doctor's life was futile.

Undertreatment

Conversely, the doctor may undertreat or prematurely give up on a patient, perceiving further treatment as futile in order to protect against feelings of despair, ineptness, or incompetence or a sense of vulnerability resulting from failure to cure. If the patient or the patient's family accentuates this feeling by berating the doctor for not doing enough and imposes guilt and a feeling of incompetence, the physician may become angry and simply give up on the patient so as not to have to give up entirely on himself. In such a situation, the doctor also fails to provide cognitive/psychologic and psychopharmacologic (including analgesic) treatment that would help the patient. In fact, failure to provide these treatments may be one of the most common forms of undertreatment in clinical medicine. Such conflicts in the physician lead to witholding of essential treatment that could enhance the patient's well-being.

Transfer of the patient to a specialist

Facing his own sense of incompetence, the physician may believe it is in the patient's best interest to obtain more optimal care by transfer to a specialist during the final phase of the patient's life. Consultations with specialists are an essential part of good medical care. However, in transferring a patient to an oncologist, cardiologist, infectious disease specialist, or other physician rather than using the specialist in a consultative or cotreatment role, the patient's doctor effectively abandons the patient at the most desperate time. While mitigating the physician's own anguish, such a transfer puts the patient in the hands of a stranger and results in the disappearance of the personal physician.

The doctor may also abandon the patient by not including the patient in rounds, by making infrequent visits, by closing off all approaches to talking about feelings and worries, and by appearing to be distracted and anxious to leave. This last reaction is often propelled by the inner tension in the physician – the feeling that if he does not leave, he will lose control, cry, break down, be less professional, and expose an all-too-human side that in the doctor's mind conveys weakness resulting from overwhelming psychologic discomfort. When feelings of despair, uncertainty, frustration, anger, or disappointment should be verbalized between the patient and the doctor to help the patient cope with these painful thoughts and affects, the doctor withdraws because of his own discomfort and feelings of failure. The doctor loses the opportunity to care for the patient – now on a psychologic level – and the patient loses a personal physician.

The C/L psychiatrist has a major role in assisting the physician, the nurse, and other caregivers to process such conflicts so as not to overtreat, undertreat, or abandon the patient. The responses in the caregivers to narcissistic injury, diminished self-esteem, loss of control (for example, crying), being angry, loss of admiration, feelings of ineptness, and pain from watching someone being extinguished before one's eyes, can all be addressed in a helpful way by the psychiatrist.

The goals of the C/L psychiatrist in these situations are to identify and acknowledge the anxieties and conflicts of the physician and other staff, to help them realize that the understandable wish to cure must be tempered by reality, and to redirect the physician's effort to a different hierarchy of care. Once these feelings and their source are understood, the physician realizes that an important task remains that could assist both the physician and the patient – the physician can do something: address the depression, anxiety, isolation, phobic response, and maladaptive reactions that are compromising the doctor–patient relationship. The physician can once again assume an active and caring role, but now on a psychologic level, and can feel capable again as the patient's physician.

Physician's words to the patient

''We are really working together in a difficult situation and doing the best we can. I think we are making important progress in helping you through this, and I am impressed at how well you are doing given the situation that you and I face. And we have faced it together. I am going to make you as comfortable as I can, and I want you to share your worries with me so you do not have to carry them by yourself. It helps to talk about your worries, and I want to hear them. It will help me take care of you better, by understanding where you are and what you are going through.''

Organ transplantation may particularly stimulate stressful conflicts because of the intensity of medical involvement and the absolute scarcity of the medical resource (the transplant organ) (Surman and Purtilo, 1992).

A liver transplant patient

A 27-year-old man with two young children developed acute liver failure following a hepatitis infection. He received a transplant; the liver failed. He received a second transplant; the liver failed. He received a third transplant; again the liver failed, and he died shortly thereafter. Should he have received a fourth transplant? Should he have had the second or even the third when other needy candidates did not have even one? The staff believed that once they had taken on this patient, they were obligated to prevent his death. After all, they had cut out his own liver. How could they then not try to replace or repair what they had done? What were their obligations to him under the Hippocratic Oath that they had taken – to ''first do no harm?'' Did they have more of an obligation to him than to the patients on whom they had not yet operated? Were other patients denied a chance, and had this unfortunate man had his fair chance with his first transplant? Can a doctor let such a patient die without trying to save him?

Was it medically futile to continue successive transplantation attempts, and was this an abrogation of distributive justice when others were denied even one opportunity?

Irrational perceptions of futility

A patient might state that "I know that everybody who has heart surgery dies. My mother died having the treatment you want me to take, and I know that I will die too." In such situations, the psychiatrist attempts to uncover the patient's fantasies that are impeding an acceptance of a medical plan for the patient's well-being, to correct the patient's erroneous ideas and beliefs regarding medical choices, and to assist the physician by demonstrating that the patient is encumbered by false beliefs. It is often not that the patient is "difficult," "passive-aggressive," or "unable to accept authority" but that the patient is convinced that the plan of the doctor will cause harm.

With regard to the dying patient, conflicts about treatment may take one of two routes: (1) the patient may refuse legitimate symptom-reducing palliative treatment because of false beliefs, or (2) the patient may demand more treatment (e.g., another operation) even though it will be of no avail and an unnecessary expenditure of medical resources. The physician may need help to ensure that his response to the patient is reality-based and, despite the difficulty of the situation, to form a medical opinion about what is needed and what is futile and present it consistently to the patient. A dilemma of distributive justice arises when resources are given futilely while needed medical interventions cannot be provided.

Fear of addicting the patient or worsening a substance abuse problem may lead the physician to deny needed narcotic medication to patients in pain (Marks and Sachar, 1973). The physician may wrongfully maintain that such a position is in the best interest of the patient and that the physician thus should not give in to the patient.

A patient with sickle cell crises

Mr. T. was a 28-year-old man who had recurrent sickle cell crises requiring many hospitalizations for stabilization and symptom relief. Each time, the staff was reluctant to prescribe the narcotic medication that the patient demanded and that from previous experience he believed he needed. Characteristically, when the house staff was reluctant to give him sufficient narcotics, he would say that he was going to kill himself. This immediately precipitated a psychiatric consultation, which invariably resulted in the psychiatrist's recommendation to adequately treat the pain associated with the crisis for 48 hours and then taper the narcotics. The patient had had eight admissions with a similar hospital course, each time with the physicians' expressing their concern that they did not want to addict the patient or go along with his "apparent substance abuse."

Conflict resolution for physicians and patient alike occurred when the psychiatrist assured the physicians that it was most unlikely that addiction would result from two days of narcotic administration. The psychiatrist reminded the physicians that on the previous seven occasions the patient had left the hospital without narcotics and had not asked for them on his subsequent visits to the sickle cell clinic.

Interpreting the patient's behavior at two levels: manifest and latent

One of the psychiatrist's major contributions to conflict resolution in the medical setting is to ferret out any unreality that may be driving decisions on the part of the physician or the patient. Inaccurate reading of the communications of patients is a common problem: "My children do not want me around and do not want to take care of a sick and dying mother, so please end my life now (''euthanize me''), and the sooner the better."

What part of this is the patient's fantasy and what part is an accurate reading of the children's feelings and conflicts? The psychologic defenses of projection, denial, repression, reaction-formation, identification with the aggressor, and identification with the victim all may influence the patient and the doctor enough to contaminate medical decision making and lead to a suboptimal decision. It is a propensity of human beings – patients and doctors alike – to have defensive maneuvers contaminate rational judgment. The psychiatrist attempts to position reality better for both.

Perhaps nowhere is this more important than in the conflict between expressed manifest mental content and latent mental wishes and longings (Strain et al. 1993). Manifest is what is said, for example, "I want to kill myself." Latent is the core unconscious feeling, which the manifest statement disguises. What is the patient really trying to say and to achieve? In the example given, it is quite possible that the patient may be simply asking for more love and understanding, but is unable to do so directly: "Will you help me through an impossible ordeal that I don't think I can manage? Will you be with me when I die? Will you keep me pain free as much as you can? Will you be there when I need you? Will you still like me if I cry, or will you hate me if you cannot make me better? Will you let me go at the right time?"

The most important effort of the psychiatrist may be to translate manifest into latent content, which is what the patient wishes and feels at bedrock (Strain et al. 1993). Decisions should be made based on an informed understanding of the latent content. A major source of error in the medical setting is the acceptance by the physician of the patient's manifest content without determining the latent, more important, wishes of the patient.

A patient with hallucinations

The patient, a well-known painter, had command hallucinations that ordered him to cut off his painting hand by chopping it with an ax on the bumper of a car for ''sins he had committed on the Astral plane 50,000 years ago.'' The patient chopped off his hand, put the severed hand in a paper bag, drove to the emergency room, and stated: ''If you try to put my hand on, I will sue you for assault and battery, cut it off again, and this time I will cut my neck as well. Throw my hand in the garbage pail! I am warning you, and for your own good you had better listen to me.'' The surgeons were profoundly influenced by what the painter said and questioned whether they should go forward with a 12-hour microsurgery reattachment (DeMuth, Strain, and Mayer-Lombardo 1983; Strain and DeMuth 1983).

The patient told the surgeons that it would be medically futile to perform 12 hours of microsurgery to reattach his severed hand. The psychiatrist learned that the patient, at a deeper, nonpsychotic level, looked forward to more painting efforts and really hoped that someone could help him. Bringing the hand to the emergency room was evidence of this wish, in contradistinction to his words. The psychiatrist began neuroleptic treatment, surgery was undertaken, fair function was restored, and the patient returned to painting. In his nonpsychotic state, he was grateful for the enormous medical efforts on his behalf, without which he could have sued for medical neglect.

The C/L psychiatrist helped the patient and his surgeons by pointing out that what appeared to be medically futile in reality was not. In the case of this painter, not operating – assessing that it was medically futile – would have been an error. Therefore, the perception of medical futility can be viewed as having two hazards: (1) doing (which goes toward no gainful end) and, (2) not doing (because action that appears as medically futile on the surface may proceed to a gainful end).

Medical decision making must be based on an understanding of the latent content, with an attempt to obtain concordance between inner unconscious feelings and conscious manifest expressions. ''I want to kill myself,'' or ''Don't do any more for me,'' or ''I want you to give me every minute I can have'' may not be what the patient fully wishes. A decision-making process based only on the patient's manifest statement does not necessarily respect the patient's autonomy. It is a decision based on incomplete and, at times, erroneous evidence of the patient's wishes. Patients' rights are not being respected by abiding by their manifest expression if it is in contradistinction to their latent wishes.

Conclusion

Medically futile situations can stimulate tremendous conflicts, both within an individual and between individuals involved in the medical situation. The psychiatrist can often assist families and patients by helping them to bear grief, guilt, and disappointment and to understand that physical helplessness does not automatically imply psychologic helplessness. Medically futile situations may in fact promote the development of psychologic mastery. Physicians too can experience psychologic growth as they turn from action at any cost to empathetic care of the whole patient, including psychologic care. Situations of perceived futility occasionally will be those in which irrational beliefs of the patient or the physician interfere with possible help. Often, a patient's manifest expression of hopelessness may mask a hidden cry for help. C/L psychiatrists, who are experienced in working in the medical setting, may be helpful in sorting through the confusion and emotional turmoil aroused by situations of real or perceived futility.

As conflicts escalate between technical advancement and scarce resources, the physician's decision-making burden also escalates. Decisions may be influenced by society, the legislature, the courts, or civil bodies. However, the doctor will remain at the nexus of difficult decisions and will continue to attempt to achieve workable compromises that respect the ethical principles of autonomy, beneficence, and distributive justice in order to provide optimal medical care. Can medical training prepare the physician to transact these diverse demands and integrate them with expert medical knowledge and personal knowledge of the patient's mental capacity, values, and wishes? Decisions involving medical futility are likely to remain to a large degree the responsibility of the doctor and the patient. Psychiatry recognizes the dilemmas involved and attempts to assist both parties by understanding complicated behavior and working to resolve the multiple conflicts that can arise.

References

DeMuth, G., Strain, J.J., and Mayer-Lombardo, A. 1983. Self-amputation and restitution. *General Hospital Psychiatry* 5:25–31.

Groves, J.E. 1979. Taking care of the hateful patient. *New England Journal of Medicine* 298:883–7.

Marks, R.M., and Sachar, E.J. 1973. Undertreatment of medical inpatients with narcotic analgesics. *Annals of Internal Medicine* 78:173–81.

Spikes, J., and Holland, J.C.B. 1975. The physician's reaction to the dying patient. In *Psychological Care of the Medically Ill: A Primer in Liaison Psychiatry.* Strain, J.J., and Grossman, S.J., eds. New York: Appleton-Century-Crofts.

Strain, J.J., Rhodes, R., Moros, D.A., and Baumrin, B. 1993. Ethics in medical practise. In *Medical Psychiatric Practise*. Stoudemire, A., and Fogel, B.S., eds., vol. 2, chap. 18, pp. 585–607. Washington, DC: American Psychiatric Press.

Strain, J.J., and DeMuth, G.W. 1983. Care of the psychotic self-amputee undergoing replantation. *Annals of Surgery* 197:210–41.

Strain, J.J., and Grossman, S.J. ed. 1975. *Psychological Care of the Medically Ill: A Primer in Liaison Psychiatry.* New York: Appleton-Century-Crofts.

Surman, O.S., and Purtilo, R. 1992. Reevaluation of organ transplantation criteria – allocation of scarce resources to borderline candidates. *Psychosomatics* 33:202–12.

11

Ethics committees and end-of-life decision making

ALICE HERB, J.D., LL.M., AND
ELIOT J. LAZAR, M.D.

End-of-life decision making, an often sad and painful process, can be need-lessly complicated by the perception that ethical dilemmas are an inevitable part of the process and necessarily result in a power struggle between patients, their families, and physicians. Ethical dilemmas do not arise in every end-of-life situation. More often, patients survive or die with little hint of an ethical problem. Typically, ethical dilemmas surface in that small number of cases in which there is genuine disagreement between the patient and the physician, between the family and the physician, among members of the family, or among members of the health care team who question the efficacy or appropriateness of continued aggressive treatment. In recent years, insti-tutional ethics committees have increasingly become the forum for the res-olution of these dilemmas. Therefore, the process of end-of-life decision making and the committee's role as consultant and mediator in the deliber-ation and resolution of these ethical dilemmas need to be better understood.

The role of ethics committees

In the context of clinical ethics, very few cases present true dilemmas. More often than not, the problem lies in poor communication between the parties, misinformation, denial of the seriousness of the illness, or reluctance to dis-cuss the issues candidly. In some instances, ethical concerns need to be sub-ordinated to prevailing law. For example, when a Jehovah's Witness refuses to accept blood transfusions or blood products, the law is clear that the pa-tient's wishes must be respected. More often, confounding ethical dilemmas involve the withholding or withdrawal of life-sustaining treatment from an incapacitated patient at the end of life. Often, the patient's preferences are not clearly known, or the patient's or family's personal values are in direct

110

conflict with standard medical practice. At the bedside, however, the dilemma is not who shall live and who shall die but rather what is in the best interest of the patient, taking into account the patient's personal values, the physician's perception of professional ethics and responsibility, and existing law.

Petitioning the courts to resolve these issues can prove to be costly and time consuming. The court experience can also be distasteful because it polarizes the participants' positions, each side mobilizing its arguments to advance its objectives. It can also be argued that these thorny issues should not be decided by judges who have no special medical training or knowledge. Indeed, in the landmark case of *In Re Quinlan* (1976), the court drew attention to the role that institutional ethics committees could perform in such heart-wrenching dilemmas. The President's Commission (1983) also promoted the idea that ethical dilemmas ought to be decided in the clinical setting and developed ideal standards for such deliberations.

An ethics committee whose members represent different disciplines but are not personally involved in the specific case would appear to provide a readily accessible forum where all parties can be heard, information concerning diagnosis, prognosis, and treatment options can be clarified, ethical and legal implications can be explained, and solutions can be explored. The ethics committee's role, however, in providing consultation and mediation is itself contentious. Many maintain that ethics committee members are not sufficiently schooled in the abstract philosophical principles of ethics to be able to identify the issues and provide appropriate guidance in such sensitive matters (Blake 1992; Hoffman 1993). Questions of cultural diversity, resource allocation, and the effect of managed care are seen as complicating the discussions in individual situations. Ethics committees can play a useful role in end-of-life decision making, but their effectiveness often depends on the commitment of the membership, the members' willingness to be educated, the availability of educational resources, the leadership qualities of the chairperson, and perhaps most important, institutional support for the process and authority of ethics committee case consultation (Sundelson 1993).

Ethics committee structure

Ethics committees in acute care facilities are as varied as the institutions in which they are located. However, they tend to share common characteristics of composition and purpose. They are multidisciplinary, typically including physicians, nurses, social workers, and administrators. Bioethics consultants, clergy, community representatives, and attorneys are frequently recruited as well. In purpose, the committee's function is usually threefold: education, policy review and development, and case review and consultation (Ross 1986).

Although institutional ethics committees may appear to be quite similar, the differences among them are usually rooted in the culture of the institution, which affects the potential power and effectiveness of the committee. Historically, ethics committees have been formed in a variety of ways: by a group of physicians or other health care providers or both who decide that they need a forum in which to discuss and resolve ethical issues, by the medical board, or by administration. Spurred in part by accreditation standards set by the Joint Commission on the Accreditation of Healthcare Organizations (JCAHO) (1996), ethics committees have become familiar fixtures at most acute care facilities. However the committee is created, it must have both administrative and medical support to achieve any degree of success. At its inception, determining whether the committee will report to the medical board or to the administration may depend on who initiated the concept of an institutional ethics committee, as well as on the internal politics of the institution. In a facility in which the physicians dominate and espouse a commitment to ethics as a part of patient care and empowerment, the committee is well served to report to the medical board. The reverse would apply where the administration is securely at the helm and commits its support.

If the committee is created at the behest of the institution, the intent of that administration is of paramount importance. Is the intent merely paper compliance to satisfy an upcoming accreditation site visit? A committee designed to place its imprimatur on administration policies and actions? An independent body that has the necessary institutional support and authority to make recommendations on policy and procedure? If the committee is a creation of the medical board, the questions are similar. For committees formed by staff initiative, whatever their professional discipline, the first order of business is to enlist institutional or medical board support or both. In assessing the potential effectiveness of an ethics committee, the committee most likely to succeed is an independent entity, sanctioned by the administration and not dependent on professional staff acceptance. Even the most elegant articulation of principle, policy, and procedure will be useless unless the institutional power structure is willing to consider and usually accept the committee's recommendations and proposals and to support its educational and case consultation initiatives.

Another important element of committee strength is leadership. When a committee is formed by interested professionals, the leadership is most likely to be selected by the participants. When it is created by either the administration or the medical board, the chairperson may be determined before the committee is organized. The selection of the chairperson sends an unmistakable message. If that person is respected professionally, has espoused an interest in ethics, and is perceived as being influential, attention is likely to be paid to the work of the committee. In addition, a committed, knowledgeable, and able leader sets the tone and the agenda for the committee.

Individual members of the committee can also make an enormous difference. Although all committees are multidisciplinary, varied representation alone is not enough. Each member's commitment, dedication, desire to learn, and willingness to consider and reflect on difficult issues are critical. The presence of a trained bioethicist is usually helpful, as it facilitates members' education and helps to frame the issues. Members trained in mediation techniques can make valuable contributions by using their skills in conflict resolution (Gibson 1994; Dubler and Marcus 1994). Attorneys, risk managers, and administrators contribute yet another perspective, although many find their presence on a committee provocative or controversial. Community members are often essential in representing the concerns of the patient population and encouraging sensitivity to cultural diversity. Participation of clergy varies among institutions from full membership to an ''as needed'' basis to not at all. It is important for the committee to distinguish between religious law and established secular principles of ethics.

Although ethics committees in long-term care facilities may bear many similarities to such committees in acute care facilities, the power structure and the substantive issues discussed are usually quite different. The focus in this chapter is principally on ethics committees in acute care institutions.

Ethics committee functions

If a committee takes on the three-part function of education, policy review/development, and case review, the first item on its agenda is self-education. Often, members are interested in ethics but have had no formal training or education in bioethics or clinical ethics. Thus, it is incumbent on the committee to plan orientation programs and educational seminars to teach the members the basic principles of ethics. A bioethicist who is a member of or a consultant to the committee can facilitate this process, which should be ongoing to update information and to educate new members. The educational function should gradually expand to include providers and other hospital staff and, finally, should form an outreach program to patients, families, and community.

Policy review and development may be the principal business of the committee early in its existence. The care and attention invested in updating and creating policies responsive to ethical issues can be educationally rewarding and bring greater insight to the membership. The process builds credibility and gives the committee visibility throughout the institution. Policy review and development are also important functions in an institution aspiring to conform to the highest standard set by JCAHO. Most facilities are appropriately concerned about the JCAHO ethics standards since ethics has become increasingly prominent in JCAHO's accreditation surveys. The ethics committee's role in the policy-making schema must be determined at the outset. Policies subject to approval by multiple bureaucratic layers or detached administrators can seriously impair the function of the committee. Policies routinely vetoed, significantly amended, or returned for substantial revision can severely undermine the credibility of the committee.

Case review is the third task of an ethics committee. Some committees limit their activities to retrospective case analysis, which can provide guidance for current and future similar situations. Committees that assume responsibility for current case consultation are also likely to be designated to mediate conflict resolution within the facility. For example, in many hospitals, the ethics committee serves as a mediator when disputes arise concerning do not resuscitate (DNR) orders.

In the ongoing work of the committee, these three functions – education, policy review/development, and case review – tend to become intermeshed. Self-education is enhanced by policy and case considerations, policy revision becomes more ethically relevant and appropriate as the committee gains experience, and case review benefits from a more educated membership.

Ethics committees and end-of-life decision making

This function is best discussed in the context of a specific case.

A woman with diabetes and hypertension
O.P. is an 87-year-old woman with a history of diabetes and hypertension. Brought to the emergency room by a neighbor, she complained of chest pain and had difficulty breathing. She was admitted, intubated, and placed on a ventilator. By the time her daughter, L.M., arrived at the hospital, O.P. was disoriented and confused. She had neither a health care proxy nor a living will, but L.M. insisted that her mother had never wanted ''extraordinary'' measures taken if she became seriously ill and wanted her mother withdrawn from the ventilator. O.P.'s son, D.P., who came the next day, was equally adamant that everything be done for his mother. The hospital physicians

maintained that they needed time to fully evaluate O.P.'s condition and were uncertain whether they could legally disconnect the ventilator.

O.P.'s case is a prototype that occurs with some frequency at acute care facilities and is used here to illustrate both the process of referral to an ethics committee and the substantive content of committee deliberations. In this scenario, seemingly irreconcilable patient-care decision-making issues arise that the physicians and health care team are unable to settle. However, an ethics committee can be an effective mechanism for resolving the conflicts and facilitating informed decision making.

In O.P.'s case, the providers are faced with the difference of opinion between brother and sister as well as with their own discomfort with disconnecting the ventilator. The providers would appropriately meet with family members first before making a referral to the ethics committee. Referrals occur when the patient or, as in this case, the family and providers are unable to agree on the patient's care or when the request to withhold or withdraw life-sustaining treatment raises ethical or legal uncertainties for the providers.

The pathway by which a dilemma may reach an ethics committee varies from facility to facility: policy and procedure may require prior administrative intervention, or a bioethicist may first attempt to resolve the issues at the bedside. If these attempts fail, the process of referral to the ethics committee usually follows a standard procedure (Ross 1986). The referral is usually made by one of the participants. The committee chairperson may then designate several members of the committee to form an ad hoc subcommittee to consult and make recommendations or to mediate and resolve the issues. Policy may require that the subcommittee either report to or seek approval from the full committee. Some committees have standing subcommittees whose specific task is case consultation.

Following this model in O.P.'s case, subcommittee members would confer with the clinicians and gather all available information concerning the patient and her condition before inviting the parties to participate in a meeting. The agenda for this first and possibly only meeting would be to focus on eliciting all relevant information about O.P. and her condition: the treatment options and providers' recommendations, the family's understanding of the patient's condition, preferences, and values, and an explanation of the ethical/legal implications. This meeting may present the first opportunity for the family and providers to speak freely and without interruption or haste, and care should be taken to put the patient or family or both at ease. It is also an opportunity to address any misinformation, misapprehension, or personal bias. If the physician in charge of O.P.'s case had never treated her before, the family might be able to furnish a more detailed medical history. If the attending physician had known her for a period of time, the physician's knowledge of the patient may be a valuable contribution.

At the outset, the subcommittee's purpose – the elucidation and resolution of perceived conflicts – should be explained in a manner that will encourage participants to freely ask questions and explore uncertainties. A brief presentation of the potential ethical and legal implications serves to inform the family and frame the discussion. The physician's medical report on the patient's diagnosis, prognosis, and current status becomes the starting point of the discussion. Explanation and reiteration may be necessary so that family members are able to understand fully the medical assessment. Since O.P. has been hospitalized for only a short time, the family may need to hear that there is still uncertainty about the diagnosis and the patient's prognosis and mental status. It is critical that O.P.'s mental status be determined because she may be able to express her own wishes to committee members during periods of clarity. O.P. may not have the capacity to decide on a treatment plan but may be capable of deciding who should make those decisions for her.

With the scant information presented about O.P. thus far, many questions need to be asked. What were the discussions between O.P. and her daughter, L.M.? What did O.P. mean by "extraordinary?" Was her statement specific to her current condition? Can this conversation be considered an expression of self-determination? Does it apply in this set of circumstances? Did O.P. also discuss her wishes with her son, D.P.? Are the best interests of the patient being considered, as the patient is incapacitated? The legal considerations can vary from state to state; for example, if the patient is hospitalized in New York State, "clear and convincing" evidence of the patient's wishes would have to be established (*In re Eichner* 1981). Additional information is essential to frame the relevant ethical and legal issues. Good decision making rests on a thorough understanding of all relevant factual information.

Another major focus for the committee would be an inquiry into the person O.P. is – her personal and medical history, living arrangements, religious beliefs, and personal values. The family would be asked if they could recall any conversations that they had with her about her fears or expectations if she were to become seriously ill and to describe her past response to illness in the family, among her friends, or in cases publicized in the media. In the course of piecing together a detailed profile of O.P., the ethical/legal issues will begin to emerge.

The portrait drawn of O.P. may indicate that before this incident, O.P. had lived alone, taking care of her own needs with minimal assistance from her daughter. Her husband's death may have been a defining event, prompting her to express her fears to her daughter. She may have feared that if she were to become seriously ill, she would lose her independence and no longer be able to live on her own. Worse yet, "extraordinary" means would be used to keep her "alive by machines," just as her husband had been. L.M. may admit that although her mother had repeatedly attempted to raise these issues with her, she tended to avoid more substantive discussions. D.P., never involved in his mother's daily life, may have been unaware of O.P.'s concerns.

One clear ethical issue for the subcommittee to consider is O.P.'s attempts to assert her autonomy in her exchanges with her daughter or perhaps with other family members or friends. Exploring the details surrounding the illness and death of O.P.'s husband may elicit more specific information about what "extraordinary" and "machines" meant to O.P.. However, since she did not leave instructions specifically refusing life-sustaining treatments, such as respirator support or dialysis, the uncertainty of her prognosis presents another issue for discussion. If it is unclear whether O.P. will be ventilator dependent or require dialysis, the providers' need for more time to stabilize the patient and conclude their workup is an important factor. With the patient's preferences (if they can be determined) or best interests central to the discussion, a waiting period would allow the physicians to conclude their medical evaluation before making any final decisions about withholding or withdrawing life-sustaining treatment and to soften or even clear up the differences between L.M. and D.P. An option that would need to be discussed separately is a DNR order in the event that O.P. experiences a cardiac arrest. If the providers agree that a DNR order is appropriate and D.P. has begun to appreciate the gravity of his mother's condition and her fears, he may consent to the entry of the order.

The legal implications differ from state to state. New York State law, for example, requires "clear and convincing" evidence of the patient's wishes if life-sustaining treatment is to be withheld or withdrawn. The one exception is a DNR order, which may be entered by a surrogate or based on a narrow, state-defined standard of medical futility. Thus, in New York State, in the absence of an advance directive, O.P.'s prior conversations with her daughter and others are critical in determining whether life-sustaining treatment could be withheld or withdrawn. In other states where surrogate decision makers are recognized without formal advance directives in place, the discussion may take a somewhat different course.

One remaining issue would be the physicians' discomfort at the specter of withdrawing the ventilator and allowing the patient to die. For this discussion, the family members should be excused so that the providers can speak more candidly. If the providers are uncertain about the legality of the withdrawal of treatment or maintain, erroneously, that there is a legal distinction between withholding and withdrawal of treatment, their perceptions and sensibilities should be addressed. A brief explanation of the ethical and legal principles may allay their concerns. If the discomfort, however, is rooted in a physician's personal belief system, the physician should be given the option to refer the case to another physician if the decision to withdraw the ventilator goes forward.

The recommendation to postpone any definitive decisions has many advantages, particularly in a case with so much factual uncertainty. First, O.P.'s diagnosis and prognosis remain uncertain. O.P. may rally and regain the capacity to make some decisions. Completion of diagnostic procedures and continued patient monitoring will have enabled the physicians to fully evaluate her condition and to assess her prognosis. L.M. and D.P. would have an opportunity to reflect on and discuss the possible options between themselves, with other family members, and with clergy or other spiritual counselors, if desirable.

A subsequent meeting, if needed, would have a more focused agenda. The discussion would now center on the decisions that can be made based on the likely outcome of O.P.'s illness. Should the medical assessment indicate that O.P. will require life-sustaining treatment indefinitely, the most successful outcome would be for the family members, fully aware that the decision is theirs, to agree to do what is legally possible and ethically in keeping with their mother's wishes, if established, or in her best interests. The physicians' recommendations may include several options: the DNR order is to remain in force, but no other treatment is to be withdrawn or withheld; dialysis is to be withheld, the DNR is to remain in force, but ventilator support is to continue; all aggressive treatment is to be withheld or withdrawn and O.P. is to be allowed to die. With the legal and ethical issues once again clearly defined, the family should be able to make informed decisions.

The effectiveness of an ethics committee lies in creating a climate in which the participants are encouraged to think about their common interest – the best interest of the patient – rather than struggle to exercise their individual rights or assert their own values. By recognizing that each participant is invested in the patient's welfare, anger and hostility can usually be diffused. In this more relaxed atmosphere, family members and providers would be better able to understand and consider the actual circumstances and each other's viewpoints. L.M. may see that her insistence on withdrawing the ventilator was premature, and her brother may realize that his mother's preferences should have priority. The physicians, no longer feeling pressured to take precipitous action, may be more accepting of a decision to withdraw treatment. It is this conciliatory mediation process that brings about a successful outcome and requires sensitivity, impartiality, and patience on the part of the ethics committee members.

Much of the success or failure of committee deliberations depends on the reasonableness of family and providers. If L.M. and D.P. remain intransigent or if the physicians do not moderate their positions, mediation may become impossible and, as occurred recently in *Gilgunn v. Massachusetts General Hospital* (1995), judicial intervention may be sought (see discussion in Capron 1995). However, the question would remain whether the committee had exerted its best effort to accommodate and address the circumstances.

Consider O.P.'s case with a different set of facts. A deeply religious woman, she had suffered from severe heart disease and diabetes for many years. This latest episode caused irreversible neurologic damage, and she lapsed into deep coma. The physicians believe that if O.P. were to experience cardiac arrest, resuscitation attempts would be futile. Moreover, the physicians believe strongly that requiring them to perform CPR on O.P. would violate their professional code of ''do no harm,'' as the burdens of CPR to O.P. far outweigh the benefits. The daughter, L.M., however, insists that O.P., in keeping with her religious beliefs, would want ''everything done'' and refuses to consider a DNR order. The other family members, though less vociferous, agree that L.M. is the appropriate spokesperson for her mother and the family.

The ethics committee would be confronted with the task of mediating between competing principles, professional ethics versus patient self-determination. Disagreement between the family and the physicians may indeed have already resulted in hostility. The committee's role here would be to facilitate communication and the exchange of information. L.M. would be encouraged to have a religious advisor or other family members accompany her to the meeting. In a neutral atmosphere, L.M. could be assured that respiratory support, dialysis, and nutrition/hydration would not be withdrawn from her mother at this point. The issue of DNR could then be precisely defined, allowing physicians to explain why they believe that CPR would be futile and, therefore, inappropriate. L.M. would also be informed that resuscitation attempts involve aggressive measures, which inevitably injure a patient in a state as fragile as is O.P. and that arrest will probably occur repeatedly before death. L.M. may need time to realize what resuscitation attempts would mean. Yet that reality may still clash with the patient's religious convictions.

In turn, L.M. would be encouraged to talk about her mother's religious beliefs. The clergyperson, if present, may confirm L.M.'s interpretation or may clarify the religious position, or L.M. may reveal that when her father was terminally ill, her mother had refused to consider a DNR order because of her firm belief in the sanctity of life. The committee may be unable to achieve a meeting of the minds but would seek to foster mutual respect among the participants. Thus, the physician may be persuaded to honor the patient's wishes and attempt resuscitation, and L.M. may begin to accept that the physicians must ultimately be able to stop the intervention if indeed it is hopeless.

An outcome that may not fully satisfy either side may be the best possible under the circumstances, yet even if an acceptable solution cannot be found and judicial intervention is sought, the committee's work may be a valuable contribution. If it can be assumed that the family and providers submitted to the consultation/mediation process in good faith, each side would, it is hoped, appreciate the sincere anguish experienced by the other.

Beyond the enumerated functions that ethics committees undertake, an ethics committee in an acute care facility has enormous potential value. Its mere presence announces to the institution's population that ethical issues arise in patient care and that these issues should be addressed. Committee members, rather than academicians or other experts, working alongside their peers, can more easily heighten awareness that advance directives, informed consent, refusal of treatment, and confidentiality mean more than abstract principles or obligatory pieces of paper. Slowly and perhaps subtly, ethics committees can become a positive influence in changing institutional think-ing. The need for such a change is perhaps best borne out by a recent study conducted by the SUPPORT Principal Investigators (1995), which showed that patients' wishes are overwhelming misunderstood or ignored by physi-cians even when they had signed advance directives or otherwise conveyed their preferences. In too many cases in which the patient should make end-of-life decisions, the matter is never discussed. However, in an atmosphere in which ethical principles become part of the institutional lexicon, patients' rights to autonomous decision making may be more readily acknowledged. The existence of an ethics committee may be a major factor in improving this situation.

Conclusion

The value of ethics committees should be assessed in a broader context than their role in facilitating or mediating end-of-life decision making. Unques-tionably, the effectiveness or acuity of many committees may be less than optimal, and committees primarily composed of professional staff may lack the necessary objectivity. However, the better argument, it would appear, is that these same professionals are experienced in medical affairs, are on site and thus readily accessible to patients, families, and clinicians, can respond immediately to emergent situations, and do not add to costs. As the role of ethics committees in providing consultation and mediation is more widely accepted, educational resources and consulting services to assist ethics committees are bound to expand. Indeed, even now, many regional networks have been formed where ethics committee members can attend seminars, ask questions, and voice their concerns. Although it is always important to strive for the ideal, it is equally important to recognize that the ideal is achieved, if ever, stepwise over time. Ethics committees learn with experience, and patients, families, clinicians, and institutions can only benefit from this process.

References

Blake, D.C. 1992. The hospital ethics committee: Health care's moral conscience or white elephant? *Hastings Center Report* 22 (Jan–Feb):6–11.

Capron, A. M. 1995. Abandoning a waning life. *Hastings Center Report* 25 (July–Aug):24–6.

Dubler, N.N., and Marcus, L.J. 1994. *Mediating Bioethical Disputes. A Practical Guide.* New York: United Hospital Fund of New York.

Gibson, J. McI. 1994. Mediation for ethics committees: a promising process. *Generations* Winter: 58–60.

Hoffman, D.E. 1993. Evaluating ethics committees: a view from the outside. *Milbank Quarterly* 71:677–701.

JCAHO Accreditation Manual for Hospitals. 1996. Patient Rights and Organization Ethics. Standards I:3543.

President's Commission for the Study of Ethical Problems in Medicine and Research. 1983. *Deciding to Forego Life-Sustaining Treatment.* Washington, DC: U.S. Government Printing Office.

Ross, J.W. 1986. *Handbook for Hospital Ethics Committees.* pp. 31–43. Chicago, IL: American Medical Association.

Sundelson, E.B. 1993. There must be a way . . . defining a role for ethics committees in health care decision making. *Trends in Health Care, Law & Ethics* 8: 45–8.

SUPPORT Principal Investigators. 1995. A controlled trial to improve care for seriously ill hospitalized patients. The Study to Understand Prognoses and Preferences for Outcomes and Risks of Treatment (SUPPORT). *Journal of the American Medical Association* 274:1591–8.

Statutes and cases

In re Eichner 52 N.Y. 2d 363, 438 N.Y.S. 2d 266, 420 N.E. 2d 64, *cert. denied,* 454 U.S. 858 (1981)

Gilgunn v. Massachusetts General Hospital, No. 92–4820 (Mass. Super. Ct. Civ. Action Suffolk Co. April 21, 1995).

In re Quinlan 70 N.J. 10, 355 A.2d 647, *cert. denied sub nom Garger v. New Jersey*, 429 U.S.922, 50 L Ed. 2d 289, 97 S. Ct. 319 (1976), *overruled in part, In re Conroy*, 98 N.J. 321, 486 A. 2d 1209 (1985).

12

The economics of futile interventions
DONALD J. MURPHY, M.D.

Futile interventions are usually expensive. Few dispute this. The question is whether limits on futile interventions will lead to significant savings. Some believe that the modest savings from futile intervention policies are not worth the burdens of these policies. Why change our ethics, law, and guidelines for medical decision making when truly futile interventions are so rare?

In this chapter, I argue that the actual cost savings of limiting futile interventions are small, but the potential cost savings are great if we consider futility in a larger context. The futile intervention debate is one of the main arenas in which our society is experiencing a cultural shift. We need to make the transition – painfully and slowly – from the rugged individualism that formed our country to a more communitarian ethic that will help us survive (and perhaps thrive) in the next century.

I consider the cost savings associated with futile interventions at three levels. First, I will review the cost savings of futile interventions that have been documented to date. Second, I consider the cost savings when we expand the futile intervention debate to include inappropriate interventions. Defining inappropriate interventions will require a change in doctors' and patients' attitudes about care near the end of life. These attitude changes could lead to significant cost savings. Third, I argue that a fundamental change in our culture is essential to control health care costs. Before considering the cost savings at these three levels, I briefly review the economics of marginally effective interventions, of which futile interventions is a prototype.

The economics of marginally effective interventions
For most health care measures, cost effectiveness is determined by the cost to treat many in order to achieve one successful outcome. Several intensive care therapies illustrate this point. First, consider intensive care for a pa-

tient with diabetic ketoacidosis. Assume that the average cost is $6,000 for two days in the hospital – one day in the intensive care unit (ICU) and one day on the ward. Since this therapy is almost universally successful, the cost required to achieve one survivor is approximately $6,000. If patients with diabetic ketoacidosis live an average of 30 years after a stay in intensive care, the cost per year of life saved is roughly $200 ($6,000 divided by 30). Hemodialysis is another example for which the success rate is essentially 100%. The cost for one year of life saved is the cost of providing dialysis to one patient for one year. This was approximately $50,000 in 1995. Both figures, $200 and $50,000, are reasonable given the standard of care in 1995.

Next, consider a therapy for which the survival rate is approximately 50%. Mechanical ventilation for a patient with AIDS who has a life-threatening infection is an example. The cost per survivor in this situation would be the total cost of treating two such patients. This cost may range from $20,000 to $60,000. Let us say $50,000. Assume the survivors live an average of 2 years after the stay in intensive care. The cost per year of life saved is, therefore, $25,000 ($50,000, the total cost, divided by 2, the number of years lived). This is a reasonable figure even though the survival rate is 50%.

Finally, consider an intervention for which the survival rate is 1% or less. Cardiopulmonary resuscitation (CPR) for nursing home residents with advanced dementia is a good example (Applebaum, King, and Finucane 1990; Awoke, Mouton, and Parrott 1992). Assume the survival to hospital discharge rate is 1%. In order for one person to survive, 100 similar patients must be treated. The total cost to achieve one successful outcome, therefore, is the cost for the 100 patients. Assume that the cost averages $4,000 per patient (this number is low because many of these patients will die after paramedics take them to the emergency room, and they will not receive intensive care). Also assume that the one survivor lives for one year. The total cost for one year of life saved (i.e., the marginal cost effectiveness ratio) is still $400,000 (Murphy and Matchar 1990).

It is evident that the number that must be treated to obtain one successful outcome is one of two major considerations. The other is the cost of the treatment (or whatever health care measure). A treatment (or screening test) that is very inexpensive may be cost effective even though thousands of patients receive the treatment in order to yield one successful outcome. Conversely, a treatment that is very expensive may not be cost effective even though the number that must be treated for one successful outcome is small. Although this discussion suggests that there is general agreement as to what is cost effective and what is not, we do not have a public consensus and have only begun a public dialogue (Murphy, Povar, and Pawlson 1994).

The actual cost savings from futile intervention policies

The direct savings from futile intervention policies are unlikely to be significant. Both clinical experience and recent studies support this claim. With few exceptions (e.g., continued CPR for failed out-of-hospital cardiac arrest), health care providers rarely provide care that all would consider futile. Returning to the example of CPR for demented nursing home residents, it is in fact rare that we provide CPR for severely demented nursing home residents (Finucane et al. 1991). A policy limiting CPR for such patients would be unlikely to save much at all. Open for debate is the question as to when continued intensive care is futile.

As director of Guidelines for the Use of Intensive Care in Denver (GUIDe), now called Colorado Collective for Medical Decisions (Murphy and Barbour 1994), I have had the opportunity to learn about many of the futile intervention cases in the Denver metropolitan area. I would estimate that, on average, hospital ethics committees deal with three to four futile interventions a year. Of course, there may be many more cases in which continued intensive care seems inappropriate but is not clearly seen as futile. Proscribing continued intensive care for this limited number of patients is unlikely to save significant sums.

An analysis by Teno et al. (1994b) from the Study to Understand Prognoses and Preferences for Outcomes and Risks of Treatments confirms that the economic savings from futile intervention policies would be modest. Of the 4,301 patients they studied, 115 (2.7%) had an estimated chance of two-month survival of $\leq$ 1%. The total hospital charges for these 115 patients was $8.8 million. By limiting life support in accord with a strict 1% futility guideline, as suggested by Schneiderman, Jecker, and Jonsen (1990), 199 of 1,688 hospital days (11.8%) would be forgone (Teno et al. 1994b). The estimated savings in hospital charges would be $1 million. Although this is not a trivial amount, these savings may not justify the anguish caused by futile intervention policies.

A study by Cohen, Lambrinos, and Fein (1993) gives us the best estimate of the cost of a year of life saved for patients who receive what could be considered futile interventions. They reported that of 22 patients whose age in years plus duration of mechanical ventilation in days totaled 100 or greater, only 2 survived hospitalization. The cost per year of life saved in this subset of patients was $181,308 in 1985–7 dollars. One of the patients was discharged to a nursing home, had multiple hospital readmissions, and died four and one-half years later. The other patient died at home months after hospital discharge.

The cost savings from limiting inappropriate intensive care

It is evident that cost savings from futile intervention policies would be modest at best. Suppose we consider limiting inappropriate interventions (not just futile interventions) for people who are near the ends of their lives. By inappropriate interventions, I mean medical interventions for which, all things considered (e.g., severity of illness, life expectancy, quality of life, cost of acute care, cost of long-term follow-up), the burdens outweigh the benefits based on a public consensus. Futile interventions, in contrast, are determined by only one factor, the patient's prognosis.

Would the cost savings from limiting inappropriate interventions be significant? An analysis by Emanuel and Emanuel (1994) suggests that the cost savings would be relatively small. They make the following claims. First, it will be difficult to reduce the amount spent for the last six months of peoples' lives because we cannot accurately predict when people will die. Second, the wider use of advance directives is unlikely to produce dramatic cost savings. Third, hospice care is not much less expensive than conventional care. Thus, the wider use of hospice is unlikely to save much. The Emanuels estimate that, under the best case assumptions (if every American who died had executed an advance directive, refused aggressive care at the end of life, and elected to receive hospice care at home), we could save 3.3.% ($29.7 billion) of the $900 billion going to health care. I would like to point out that a 3% savings on the health care budget is not a trivial amount. Many successful businesses would consider a 3% cost reduction quite significant.

My response is, first, it is true that we cannot accurately predict when someone will die (Forster and Lynn 1988). We cannot prospectively identify the last six months of someone's life. On the other hand, we are not completely ignorant. For many chronically ill patients with superimposed acute illness, we can predict their likelihood of surviving six months with a fair degree of accuracy (Knaus et al. 1995). For most chronically ill patients (i.e., patients with end-stage heart, lung, liver, or brain disease) who are stable, we have a good idea when they are reaching their last two to three years of life. If, then, we could focus on the cost savings in the last two to three years of life (not just the last six months) and we could learn to live with the inherent inaccuracies in the science of prediction, we could realize considerable savings. Of course, there is a price to this change in mindset. Someone will die nine months (or perhaps even two years) before they would have died with more aggressive care. I believe many chronically ill seniors would accept this change in mindset if they could be assured that the savings would be put to good use, such as long-term care insurance, programs to alleviate loneliness in old age, better housing, or even better education for their grandchildren.

Second, I agree that wider use of advance directives will not result in dramatic savings, at least not in the current climate. However, three studies suggest that advance directives will lead to some savings (Weeks et al. 1994; Chambers et al. 1994; Maksoud, Jahnigen, and Skibinski 1993). They indicate that hospital charges are two to seven times higher for patients who die and did not have written advance directives before hospitalization than for patients who die and did have written advance directives. These three studies were retrospective chart reviews.

In contrast, Schneiderman et al. (1992) reported that the costs for medical interventions in the last month of life were the same for patients offered an advance directive and for controls (i.e., no specific plan to offer advance directives). This was a randomized, controlled trial. The largest and most robust study is the SUPPORT study (Youngner, Murphy, and Lynn 1990). Teno and the SUPPORT investigators found no significant cost savings associated with advance directives (Teno et al. 1994a; Teno et al. 1997). Interestingly, Teno et al. would have found cost savings associated with advance directives if they had limited their analyses to the use of only retrospective data among control patients in phase II of SUPPORT (Teno et al. 1997). Such retrospective analyses can be misleading.

Although advance directives may not be associated with significant cost savings now, that may change. The reason is that advance directives currently do not mean as much as we would like to think. Our fantasy is that formal directives (living wills or durable powers of attorney) assure patient autonomy and that patients' preferences will be honored. Often, advance directives fail to meet this challenge. So much depends on physicians' attitudes about advance directives, their general attitudes about care near the end of life, and their role as stewards of limited resources. If the wider use of advance directives were accompanied by a major attitude change among providers and patients, we might see dramatic savings associated with advance directives. It will be interesting to see if the transition from fee-for-service to capitation will facilitate this attitude change (Morrison and Meier 1995).

Third, I believe that the Emanuels' analysis underestimates the potential cost savings from wider use of hospice or at least palliative care. The Emanuels claim that the studies reporting cost savings with hospice care are retrospective and may overestimate savings. Indeed, the latest report of cost savings associated with hospice is retrospective and is susceptible to the same biases as the other retrospective studies (Mitchell et al. 1994). However, the differences in cost are impressive. In their study of charges of hospice and nonhospice patients, Mitchell et al. (1994) reported that the median daily and total charges for hospice patients ($88 and $986, respectively) were significantly lower than charges for nonhospice patients ($999 and $7,731, respectively).

Significant savings associated with hospice care may be realized when we provide such care to many more patients than are currently eligible for hospice. My claim is that expanding the futile intervention debate to a public debate on the appropriateness of life-sustaining interventions will lead to much greater savings. Limiting inappropriate interventions could, I believe, save as much as 6% to 10% of the health care budget. Although this is speculation, I elaborate on work from the Colorado Collective for Medical Decisions (CCMD) to illustrate these points.

Over the past year, the adult intensive care subcommittee from CCMD has developed a scale to help measure inappropriate interventions. Although we cannot categorize care as either appropriate or inappropriate, we can try to measure degrees of appropriateness. After a year-long discussion, the committee decided to study six parameters: (1) premorbid life expectancy (i.e., the patient's life expectancy before the acute illness requiring hospitalization), (2) severity of the acute illness, (3) cost of treating the acute illness, (4) cost of treating chronic illnesses or long-term sequelae of the acute illness, (5) expected mental status after the patient recovers from the acute illness, and (6) the role of substance abuse (i.e., tobacco, alcohol, or illicit drugs) or high-risk behaviors in the patient's current illness. Many clinicians and ethicists believe that probability of benefit is the key factor in determining the appropriateness of treatments. I suggest that it is only one factor in this determination and that others are important, too. Consider, for example, three individuals with serious illnesses. They all have the same severity of acute illness; all have a 10% chance of surviving to discharge. One was healthy before hospitalization. Another had a moderate dementia and was ready to enter a nursing home. The third had severe dementia as well as other medical problems that gave her a life expectancy of less than a year. A dialogue with the public, using the CCMD scale or other means of discourse, may lead to a conclusion that intensive care is appropriate for the first individual and is of questionable appropriateness for the second and that hospice is appropriate for the third person (Volicer et al. 1994; Luchins and Hanrahan 1993).

Based on my discussions with patients (Murphy 1988; Murphy et al. 1994) and with professionals, I predict that professionals and laypersons will eventually agree that palliative care is, much more often than not, the appropriate response to an acute illness for patients with (1) persistent vegetative state, (2) moderate to advanced dementia, (3) chronic illness and a limited life expectancy (i.e., less than a year), (4) less than a 25% chance of surviving and very old (i.e., over 85 years), and (5) self-induced illness and no plans to correct the risky behaviors or seek treatment (e.g., the alcoholic who has refused treatment for alcoholism and experiences his fourth esophageal bleed). Furthermore, I predict that we will use palliative care earlier than we do now for patients with multiple organ system failure who have not responded to intensive care. Many patients fitting into these categories continue to receive intensive care (or life-sustaining care on the general medical and surgical wards), and it is not considered futile. Once consensus is reached that much of this care is inappropriate and practice patterns change accordingly, we will save much more than estimated by Emanuel and Emanuel (1994).

Three lines of evidence suggest that we could realize significant savings with reduction of inappropriate intensive care. The first is that the cost of care for patients who are seriously ill (i.e., APACHE II scores of 21–40) can be two to three times higher than the cost of care for patients who are the most seriously ill (i.e., APACHE II scores of > 45) (Oye and Bellamy 1991). Many types of inappropriate treatments, based on the factors listed previously and not just on severity of illness, would be associated with this middle range of severity of illness scores. The uncertainty of the prognosis leads to the prolongation of intensive care, and the costs rise accordingly.

The second line of evidence comes from a study of 1,402 consecutively admitted patients to the Stanford ICU in 1989 (Esserman, Belkora, and Lenert 1995). Esserman et al. defined potentially ineffective care (PIC) as resource use in the upper 25th percentile and survival for less than 100 days after discharge. Reduction of intensity of treatment after a prediction of PIC may save $1.8 million to $5 million per year in one hospital.

A third line of evidence is that the expenses for care during the last year of an average Medicare beneficiary's life are approximately 24% to 30% of the total Medicare budget (Lubitz and Riley 1993; Scitovsky 1994). More than 60% of these expenditures are in the three months before death (McCall 1984; Lubitz and Riley 1993; Scitovsky 1994). Again, it is the uncertainty in prognosis that leads to more extensive and costly care for this population. Once we determine the goals of medicine and appropriateness of treatments based on factors besides prognosis, we will provide more palliative care and less life-sustaining care than we currently provide. The savings associated with a more mature acceptance of our mortality (Callahan 1993) could be significant.

Why focus on futility?

Why, then, do we even talk about the economics of futile interventions if futile interventions are not where we find a lot of money? The answer is simple and, again, speculative. If our society cannot deal responsibly with futile interventions (i.e., merge good ethics, good patient care, and good economics), we have little hope of dealing responsibly with the much greater volume of inappropriate intensive care. Furthermore, we will have great difficulty dealing responsibly with any kind of marginally beneficial care. The Oregon experiment, particularly the limits on low priority services, informs us how difficult these struggles will be for our society (Eddy 1991). If our society does succeed in limiting futile interventions, we have a much greater chance of saving significant sums by limiting inappropriate and marginally beneficial care across the clinical spectrum (screening, prophylaxis, surveillance, diagnostics, and therapeutics) (Murphy, Povar, and Pawlson 1994).

The futile intervention debate is not as much about actual dollars saved as it is about values. A change in values (e.g., less individualism and a greater focus on communities and stewardship) will indeed lead to significant savings. No one can accurately estimate the dollar value at this time. It is likely to be high.

The cost saving from a cultural shift

Results from the SUPPORT study (SUPPORT Principal Investigators, 1995) suggest that we must consider a cultural shift if we are to improve care near the end of life and control the cost of dying. A fairly aggressive intervention (nurses facilitating communication about patient preferences, prognoses, and symptoms) failed to have an impact on patient–physician communication, timing of do not resuscitate (DNR) orders, reduction of inappropriate intensive care, symptom control, and reduced use of hospital resources. Lo's editorial (1995) recognized the need for a cultural change in American hospitals. I believe the cultural shift needs to occur outside the hospital walls as well as inside the ICU.

When considering shifts in our culture, we need to adjust our mindset. Rather than focus on data and hypotheses found in the literature (medical, ethical, legal, or economic), we should look at the signs of the times. For the moment, let us try to quiet the scientists and philosophers within and simply observe our culture. I suggest that we look at a best-selling book, a trial that filled our airwaves and print media, and a political hot potato. Specifically, I would like to consider Philip Howard's book, *The Death of Common Sense* (Howard 1995), the O.J. Simpson trial, and gun control.

Howard's message is that we have allowed rules and regulations to replace good judgment. Our society is full of laws that make little or no sense. For example, streets in suburbia are 50 feet wide because the traffic engineers who wrote the codes after World War II believed that streets had to be wide enough to allow two fire engines going in opposite directions to pass each other at 50 mph. Mother Theresa's Sisters of Charity would have had to pay more than $100,000 to put an elevator in an abandoned building that they wanted to convert into a community home for 64 homeless men. The Sisters of Charity avoid the routine use of modern conveniences and do not need an elevator to provide compassionate care to the homeless. Examples abound about the death of common sense, and medicine has its share.

Consider DNR orders. I know that many purists will consider the following thought experiment an apostasy. However, I believe we should be open to the possibility that much of our preoccupation with bioethics is a result of the death (or at least dying) of common sense. Imagine a world without DNR orders. Assume that we allowed, in fact encouraged, professionals and lay-persons to use good judgment about the use of CPR. If an 85-year-old nursing home resident with advanced dementia had a cardiac arrest, no one would start CPR. I have spoken with thousands of patients, professionals, and lay-persons about this scenario. With the exception of one woman whose family was killed in the Holocaust, I have found no one who would want CPR once they understand CPR and its outcomes. Conversely, if a 50-year-old marathon runner had a cardiac arrest during a race, bystanders would start CPR and do everything possible to ensure that the man received advanced cardiac life support. I have spoken with hundreds about this scenario. With few exceptions, all would want CPR. Some would call this view biased (perhaps the preferences I elicit – with individuals or with groups – reflect my biases) and fear the loss of patient autonomy. Others would call it common sense.

Granted, many scenarios are not as clear-cut as these two extremes. However, I believe that reliance on good judgment rather than on rules and regulations would lead to better outcomes. Average CPR outcomes would certainly improve because CPR would be reserved for appropriate circumstances, and futile CPR attempts would be rare. Patients, families, and professionals would probably be more satisfied. Good judgment would allow all to maintain their integrity, and we could reduce costs.

Imagine the costs associated with (1) formal DNR policies, (2) discussions with patients and families about futile interventions, (3) legislation such as the Patient Self Determination Act, (4) ethics committee consultations about DNR orders, (5) research about DNR orders, and (6) continuing education about DNR orders. Further, imagine the costs associated with discussions, consultations, policies, research, and education about inappropriate life-sustaining care. I can only speculate that the cost of common sense is much less than the cost of a myriad of laws, rules, and regulations. The outcomes, regardless of the costs, might even favor common sense.

From an economic perspective, the O.J. Simpson trial is analogous to futile interventions in medicine. Both epitomize the wasteful use of resources. Richard Parker, a law professor at Harvard, states (1995):

The waste in our system of criminal ''justice'' – in terms of allocation of collective resources – is easy to see. Our goal is fair, accurate and effective enforcement of the law. The question is how much time and money and talent we should spend and how we should spend it. We could spend on every case the resources that will, eventually, be spent on the Simpson case. In every case, lawyers and investigators might explore every complexity, testing every bit of evidence, as elaborately as in the Simpson case. But the adversary system might then bankrupt us before the health-care system does the job.

Just as our society has difficulty with limits in medicine, we have difficulty with limits in other professions. Parker claims that a populist movement may lead to reforms in the adversary system that may limit the costs of that system. The futile intervention debate could also evolve into a populist movement that results in better control of health care costs.

The gun control debate illustrates another preoccupation (almost obsession) in our culture. We strongly resist any attempt to limit our individual rights. Do millions of National Rifle Association members who oppose all gun control laws really think that it is acceptable for a teenager to buy guns without any restrictions? I doubt it. What the NRA members are saying is – do not interfere with my right to bear arms. The focus is on individual rights, not on the health of communities. Once again, I can only speculate about the cost of protecting all individual rights. It must be high. I suspect it is every bit as high as the cost needed to build healthy communities. The outcomes, regardless of the costs, might even favor an emphasis on community and reasonable restrictions on individual rights (Callahan 1990).

These three snapshots of our culture make us uncomfortable, and they should. They tell us a lot about our soul. We have hang-ups. We do not trust common sense; instead we legislate and regulate at great expense. We do not know how to set limits; instead we waste resources at great expense. We do not focus enough on communities; instead we obsess over perceived rights for individuals at great expense.

Conclusion

The futile intervention debate is helping us overcome these hang-ups in our culture. It is helping us trust common sense, set appropriate limits, and think of communities. When we make this cultural shift, the cost savings could be substantial. We not only will reduce health care costs but also will be more likely to reduce costs associated with marginal benefits in other walks of life (e.g., law, defense, education, athletics).

The economics of futile interventions deserves more study. Our research, however, should not be limited to the work of economists, ethicists, and clinicians. If, indeed, futility serves as a cultural compass, we will need many disciplines to contribute to this debate.

References

Applebaum, G.E., King, J.E., and Finucane, T.E. 1990. The outcome of CPR initiated in nursing homes. *Journal of the American Geriatrics Society* 38:197–200.

Awoke, S., Mouton, C.P., and Parrott, M. 1992. Outcomes of skilled cardiopulmonary resuscitation in a long-term-care facility: futile therapy? *Journal of the American Geriatrics Society* 40:593–5.

Callahan, D. 1990. *What Kind of Life: The Limits of Medical Progress.* New York: Simon & Schuster.

Callahan, D. 1993. *The Troubled Dream of Life.* New York: Simon & Schuster.

Chambers, C.V., Diamond, J.J., Perkel, R.L., and Lasch, L.A. 1994. Relationship of advance directives to hospital charges in a Medicare population. *Archives of Internal Medicine.* 154:541–7.

Cohen, I.L., Lambrinos, J., and Fein, I.A. 1993. Mechanical ventilation for the elderly patient in intensive care: incremental charges and benefits. *Journal of the American Medical Association* 269:1025–9.

Eddy, D.M. 1991. What's going on in Oregon? *Journal of the American Medical Association* 266:417–20.

Emanuel, E.J., and Emanuel, L.L. 1994. The economics of dying. The illusion of cost savings at the end of life. *New England Journal of Medicine* 330:540–4.

Esserman, L., Belkora, J., and Lenert, L. 1995. Potentially ineffective care: a new outcome to assess the limits of critical care. *Journal of the American Medical Association* 274:1544–51.

Finucane, T.E., Boyer, J.T., Bulmash, J., et al. 1991. The incidence of attempted CPR in nursing homes. *Journal of the American Geriatrics Society* 39:624–6.

Forster, L.E., and Lynn, J. 1988. Predicting life span for applicants to inpatient hospice. *Archives of Internal Medicine* 148:2540–3.

Howard, P.K. 1995. *The Death of Common Sense.* New York: Random House.

Knaus, W.A., Harrell, F.E., Jr., Lynn, J., et al. for the SUPPORT investigators.

1995. The SUPPORT prognostic model: objective estimates of survival for seriously ill hospitalized adults. *Annals of Internal Medicine* 122:191–203.

Lo, B. 1995. Improving care near the end of life. Why is it so hard? *Journal of the American Medical Association* 274:1634–6.

Lubitz, J.D., and Riley, G.F. 1993. Trends in Medicare payments in the last year of life. *New England Journal of Medicine* 328:1092–6.

Luchins, D.J., and Hanrahan, P. 1993. What is appropriate health care for end-stage dementia? *Journal of the American Geriatrics Society* 41:25–30.

Maksoud, A., Jahnigen, D.W., and Skibinski, C.I. 1993. Do not resuscitate orders and the cost of death. *Archives of Internal Medicine* 153:1249–53.

McCall, N. 1984. Utilization and costs of Medicare services by beneficiaries in their last year of life. *Medical Care* 22:329–42.

Mitchell, A., Hunter, D., Blackhurst, D., et al. 1994. Hospice care: the cheaper alternative. *Journal of the American Medical Association* 271:1576–7.

Morrison, R.S., and Meier, D.E. 1995. Managed care at the end of life. *Trends in Health Care, Law & Ethics* 10:91–6.

Murphy, D.J. 1988. Do-not-resuscitate orders. Time for reappraisal in long-term-care institutions. *Journal of the American Medical Association* 260:2098–101.

Murphy, D.J., and Barbour, E. 1994. GUIDe (Guidelines for the Use of Intensive Care in Denver): a community effort to define futile and inappropriate care. *New Horizons* 2:326–31.

Murphy, D.J., Burrows, D., Santilli, S., et al. 1994. The influence of the probability of survival on patients' preferences regarding cardiopulmonary resuscitation. *New England Journal of Medicine* 330:545–9.

Murphy, D.J., and Matchar, D.B. 1990. Life-sustaining therapy. A model for appropriate use. *Journal of the American Medical Association* 264:2103–8.

Murphy, D.J., Povar, G.J., and Pawlson, L.G. 1994. Setting limits in clinical medicine. *Archives of Internal Medicine* 154:505–12.

Oye R.K., and Bellamy, P.E. 1991. Patterns of resource consumption in medical intensive care. *Chest* 99:685–9.

Parker, R. 1995. The coming legal backlash. *New Republic* March 20:21–4.

Schneiderman, L.J., Jecker, N.S., and Jonsen, A.R. 1990. Medical futility: its meaning and ethical implications. *Annals of Internal Medicine* 112:949–54.

Schneiderman L.J., Kronick, R., Kaplan, R.M., et al. 1992. Effects of offering advance directives on medical treatments and costs. *Annals of Internal Medicine.* 117:599–606.

Scitovsky, A.A. 1994. "The high cost of dying" revisited. *Milbank Quarterly* 72: 561–91.

SUPPORT Principal Investigators. 1995. A controlled trial to improve care for seriously ill hospitalized patients. The Study to Understand Prognoses and Preferences for Outcomes and Risks of Treatments (SUPPORT). *Journal of the American Medical Association* 274:1591–8.

Teno, J., Lynn, J., Connors, A.F., Jr., et al. for the SUPPORT investigators. 1997. The illusion of end-of-life resource savings with advance directives. *Journal of the American Geriatrics Society.*

Teno, J.M., Lynn, J., Phillips, R.S., et al. for the SUPPORT investigators. 1994a. Do formal advance directives affect resuscitation decisions and the use of resources for seriously ill patients? *Journal of Clinical Ethics* 5:23–30.

Teno, J.M., Murphy, D.J., Lynn, J., et al. for the SUPPORT investigators. 1994b. Prognosis-based futility guidelines: does anyone win? *Journal of the American Geriatrics Society* 42:1202–7.

Volicer, L., Collard, A., Hurley, A., et al. 1994. Impact of special care unit for patients with advanced Alzheimer's disease on patients' discomfort and costs. *Journal of the American Geriatrics Society.* 42:597–603.

Weeks, W.B., Kofoed, L.L., Wallace, A.E., and Welch, H.G. 1994. Advance directives and the cost of terminal hospitalization. *Archives of Internal Medicine* 154:2077–83.

Youngner, S.J., Murphy, D.J., and Lynn, J. 1990. Decision making in SUPPORT: sentinel decisions. *Journal of Clinical Epidemiology* 43 (Suppl):67S–71S.

13

Medical futility: a legal perspective

WILLIAM PRIP, M.A., AND
ANNA MORETTI, R.N., J.D.

For the past two decades, much of the medical, ethical, and legal discussion about death and dying has focused on the right of individuals to reject treatments that only prolong the dying process. Yet if the volume of literature devoted to medical futility in recent years is any indicator, a significant number of individuals are now clamoring for the very treatments that others fought to reject.

Much of this discussion concerning medical futility comes from a medical or philosophical perspective. On the few occasions that the judicial system has addressed the subject of medical futility, it has applied the law unevenly and often without much reflection about the consequences of its rulings, leaving clinicians and patients with little guidance. Statutes that address medical futility directly are fewer still and have proved ineffective at resolving the hypothetical and real problems that the futility debate creates for clinicians and patients across the country.

In this chapter, we survey the legislation and court decisions that have specifically addressed the issues of medical futility and explore whether the established right to refuse treatment can inform the futility debate and the right to receive treatment, or whether a new set of laws and legal principles is needed.

The emergence of the futility problem

A consensus on what constitutes futile treatment remains elusive. However, conflicts over medical futility are beginning to surface as a new type of end-of-life decision-making case. As medical technology developed over the years, a standard emerged that demanded treatment at all cost without much thought to outcome. One of the consequences of this reflexive standard was the emergence of the right-to-die movement. Patients became more vocal in

136

their refusal of treatment that merely prolonged the dying process, and, eventually, advance directive statutes were enacted in every state. In effect, patients were telling physicians that, from their perspective, treatment that could not return them to an acceptable quality of life was futile.

We now have come full circle; patients and their families are challenging the physician's decision to stop life-sustaining treatment. Today, physicians assert that the treatments being requested are futile and that providing them would be contrary to the accepted standard of care for that medical situation.

Although standards of care may serve as the legal defense in medical malpractice cases, it is unclear what constitutes accepted standards of care or reasonable medical practice in the futility case scenario. Despite the availability of scientifically developed indicators of the efficacy of various medical treatments and procedures, physicians cannot consistently define futility (Curtis et al. 1995). The treatments offered to dying patients with similar prognoses may differ significantly. As there are no standards of practice that say that treatment must stop, physicians decide what is futile on a case by case basis. To date, this ad hoc approach has not been effective in creating standards of care that can be applied uniformly in the clinical setting.[1]

Is medical futility a legal issue?

Whatever one's position in the futility debate, an important question remains: Does the law offer an effective remedy for the futility problem? If the law indeed becomes the arbiter between patients and physicians in the futility debate, will a formal legal process be constructed for identifying futility, or will the courts rely on an approach similar to Justice Stewart Potter's technique for identifying obscenity: "I know it when I see it"?

Clearly, the law has had considerable influence in effecting a consensus on some contentious social issues concerning medical ethics.[2] Indeed, the

---

[1] The case of Baby Nguyen is evidence that practice variation adds to the tenuous nature of using "accepted medical standards" as the legal basis for stopping treatment. Ryan Nguyen was born with severe medical problems, including kidney failure, bowel obstruction, and brain damage. Although physicians at one hospital argued that continued aggressive treatment would only prolong his suffering, physicians at another facility were more than willing to continue aggressive treatment (Kolata 1994).

[2] For example, the consensus today that brain death is a definition of death has its roots in 1970 when the Kansas Legislature enacted a law, sponsored by a physician–legislator, that included an alternative definition to the common-law and customary method of defining death: a cessation of circulatory or respiratory function (President's Commission 1981:62). Although the new definition still relied on physicians to determine whether death had occurred – specifically, to determine if there was an "absence of spontaneous brain function" – this legal watershed undoubtedly influenced other developments, including model brain death standards issued by

138 William Prip and Anna Moretti

New Jersey Supreme Court's 1976 ruling in the Karen Ann Quinlan case provided the impetus for much of the debate about patient autonomy in end-of-life decision making for the next two decades. Not only did the notoriety of the case provide the catalyst for enactment of the nation's first living will law in California later that year (Glick 1992:53), but it undoubtedly sparked the public's interest in the issue that eventually produced a devolution of power from doctors to patients regarding end-of-life decision making. By 1982, the year the American Medical Association's Judicial Council concluded that "withholding or removing life supporting means is ethical" (President's Commission 1983:299), 13 states and the District of Columbia had already enacted advance directive laws,[3] and six appellate state courts had decided on right-to-die cases.[4] Clearly, the medical profession's standards of care have lagged behind the law in addressing the issue of a patient's right to refuse unwanted care.

However, although it may be convenient and appear expeditious to defer to the law for resolution of the futility debate, we must realize at the outset that the law governing the right of patients to refuse treatment has not been very successful in affecting the behavior of health care providers in the clinical setting. It is important to remember that even after more than two decades of litigation and legislation protecting the right of patients to refuse unwanted care, the preponderance of decision-making conflicts involving critically ill patients still results from the reluctance of the physician or health care institution to permit the forgoing of unwanted life-sustaining measures.

Legal rights in the futility debate

One can argue that the right to demand and receive medical treatment even when it is deemed medically ineffective by the attending physician is a logical extension of the right to patient autonomy.[5] This argument observes roughly the following logic: if one has the right to control one's health care by refusing medical treatment even if that decision is contrary to medical advice, one also retains the right to request and receive health care,

the American Bar Association in 1975, the National Conference of Commissioners on Uniform State Laws in 1978, and the American Medical Association in 1979 (President's Commission 1981: 117–19). Eventually, in 1980–81, all three groups settled on the Uniform Law Commissioners' "Uniform Definition of Death Act," which has been enacted in all but three states.
[3] Alabama, Arkansas, California, Delaware, Idaho, Kansas, Nevada, New Mexico, North Carolina, Oregon, Texas, Vermont, Washington, and the District of Columbia.
[4] Florida, Massachusetts, New Jersey, New York, Tennessee, and Louisiana.
[5] Proponents of the right to assisted suicide argue similarly that the right to autonomy in medical decision making encompasses the right to receive, directly or indirectly, death-inducing medications (*Compassion in Dying v. Washington* 1994).

again over a physician's objections. In essence, this position contends that the right to patient autonomy would be hollow if it were confined only to the right to refuse care – regardless of the fact that most patient self-determination laws are silent regarding the right to receive treatment. An analogous argument, although applied to effect the reverse conclusion, has been made regarding the common law doctrine of informed consent. That is, if, as in the words of the U.S. Supreme Court, the "logical corollary of the doctrine of informed consent is that the patient generally possesses the right not to consent, that is, to refuse treatment" (*Cruzan v. Director* 1990: 270), the logical corollary of the right to refuse treatment is the right to receive treatment.

Although this logic may be compelling, it is important to realize that the law underlying the right to refuse treatment does not easily transfer to the right to receive treatment. The difference between the demands "don't touch me" and "you must touch me" is dramatic. The law has almost uniformly conceded the former but has only hesitantly recognized the latter, and only in situations related to public health and safety.

The right to refuse versus the right to receive

The challenge is to determine if the patient autonomy model, as it has evolved over recent years, adequately addresses the futility question. Historically, the public readily accepted the dominance of patient autonomy over the "doctor knows best" approach to medical decision making, although it took well over a decade, beginning in 1976 with the *Quinlan* ruling, for the issue to permeate the American consciousness. Today, the right to refuse treatment is supported by a myriad of laws: all states and the District of Columbia have enacted advance directive legislation. All of the state appellate courts that have addressed the issue have found a legal right of patients to forgo life-prolonging procedures; the U.S. Supreme Court has ruled that patients have a constitutional right to be free of unwanted medical treatments, and the Congress has enacted federal legislation aimed at educating the public about their right to refuse treatment under state law.

However, the right asserted in futility cases is different. As Meisel points out, the right to refuse treatment and the right to receive treatment are, respectively, negative and positive rights (Meisel 1995:546–8). A negative right bestows on individuals a right that is protected by prohibiting others from certain behavior. The right to liberty guarantees personal freedom, for example, by prohibiting incarceration by the state without due process. In contrast, a positive right obliges others to provide a service or expend resources in order for an individual to exercise such right. Certain civil and political rights, as well as rights established by government entitlement programs and consumer protection laws, are positive rights. Thus, both the right to a trial by jury and the right to suffrage require the state to establish and support processes that guarantee these positive rights to all citizens. Similarly, consumer protection laws require that consumers be provided with nutrition information and content labels on all food products sold in the country – that is, the state establishes a positive right (to information) and obliges another private actor to fulfill the right.

Importantly, a positive right to be touched by another is only found in the area of public health and safety and is established exclusively by statute. For example, many cities and states have created rights to certain types of health care under the aegis of sound public policy, such as prenatal care for indigent mothers-to-be and immunization for children. Individuals also have the right to be touched for safety purposes in emergency situations, including the right to receive assistance from rescue squads, fire departments, and emergency medical services.

In applying the concept of negative and positive rights to the issue of patient autonomy, Meisel writes (1995:546)

A *negative* right embodies the freedom to do what one wants without interference from others. The right to refuse medical treatment is such a right. . . . The right being asserted in futility cases, by contrast, is a *positive* right. . . . In the context of medical decisionmaking, it is the freedom to have whatever medical treatment one might wish.

As a negative right, the right to refuse medical care, whether life saving or routine, is bolstered by a long legal tradition, rooted in the constitutional right to privacy and liberty and the common law right to be let alone. As early as 1891, the right to be free of unwanted touching was articulated by the U.S. Supreme Court: "No right is held more sacred, or is more carefully guarded, by the common law, than the right of every individual to the possession and control of his own person, free from all restraint or interference of others, unless by clear and unquestionable authority of law" (*Union Pacific R. Co. v. Botsford* 1891:25). Over 20 years later, Justice Benjamin Cardozo applied this thinking to medical treatments: "Every human being of adult years and sound mind has a right to determine what shall be done with his own body; and a surgeon who performs an operation without his patient's consent commits an assault, for which he is liable in damages" (*Schloendorff v. Society of New York Hospital* 1914:129–30).

In this respect, the right to refuse treatment dictates that bodily integrity must not be violated without informed consent. Indeed, to trespass upon the person without consent is generally considered a tortious act that is compensable in damages. Over the years, penalties for nonconsensual touching in the medical setting have been articulated in numerous cases.[6] Even when a treatment is beneficial, the courts have frowned on nonconsensual touching. For example, an Ohio appeals court declared, ''[a] physician who treats a patient without consent commits a battery, even though the procedure is harmless or beneficial'' (*Leach v. Shapiro* 1984:1051).

In contrast, the right to receive treatment is not supported by a similar historic foundation. Indeed, the federal judiciary has been reluctant to find a constitutional right that requires the state or other individuals to provide services or expend resources or both to safeguard an individual's claim to such right. Even through the various tort remedies in common law that better govern the relations between private actors, the right asserted in futility cases is not firmly settled.

A recent law review note asserted that elements in the theory of negligence, specifically, the concept of a legal duty to act, can be used to penalize physicians who unilaterally deny health care to their patients (Mordarski 1993: 765).

In a case in which a patient is dependent on a life support system, the physician would have duty to act as a reasonable physician would act when dealing with that patient. If the physician were to terminate the life support system against the wishes of the family, the family would have to convince a jury that a reasonable physician, in the same circumstances, would not have terminated the life support.

This line of argument was put to test in a recent law suit (*Gilgunn* 1995) brought by the daughter of a patient who died as a result of the withdrawal of ventilator support and the withholding of cardiopulmonary resuscitation (CPR). However, a jury refused to find the defendants (the hospital, the physician who wrote the do not resuscitate, DNR, order, and the head of the ethics committee) negligent because the jury believed the treatments requested by the daughter were ''futile.''

---

[6] See, for example, *Mohr v. Williams* (1905) (allowing recovery of damages for assault and battery against a physician who operated on the left ear of patient who only consented to surgery on the right ear); *Schmeltz v. Tracy* (1935) (permitting assault and battery charges against a physician who removed moles not consented to during a consent to acne procedure); *Chouinard v. Marjani* (1990) (accepting negligence and intentional assault charges for performance of bilateral surgery when patient only consented to surgery on one breast); *Fox v. Smith* (1992) (acknowledging battery claim against a physician for removal of intrauterine device without consent from a patient undergoing another procedure); *Perkins v. Lavin* (1994) (permitting assault and battery claim against a hospital for the administration of a blood transfusion against patient's explicit instructions); *Cohen v. Smith* (1995) (allowing claims of battery and intentional infliction of emotional distress for allowing a male nurse to view and touch an unclothed female patient against patient's wishes).

Another approach to the futility debate is to consider the issue of abandonment. In general, a duty is imposed on physicians to continue to care for their patients once the patient–physician relationship has been established unless the relationship is terminated by the patient or the physician after reasonable notice to the patient. To prove that a physician abandoned a patient, however, it would be necessary to demonstrate that the physician "completely and unilaterally sever[ed] the relationship" with the patient (Meisel 1995:39), an unlikely situation in a futility case, in which a physician, for example, may refuse to provide artificial ventilation but would likely continue various other treatments. Medical abandonment is a complex issue that, to date, has not been applied to medical futility. However, it is possible that a patient may rely on the duty of nonabandonment to request treatment from a physician with whom he or she has had a long-standing patient–physician relationship.[7]

Meisel suggests that perhaps another recourse for patients and their families requesting treatment is to argue that a contractual relationship between a physician and patient requires the patient's wishes to be honored (Meisel 1995:548). This argument, however, has not been tested in the courts.

Perhaps the right to receive treatment, then, must rely solely on statutory law, which is generally the mechanism used to establish positive rights. Indeed, because it is the only method of creating a positive right that compels another individual to touch the person exercising the right, a legal resolution of the futility debate may lie in the hands of the federal and state legislatures, although courts may be forced to rely on creative interpretations of existing statutes in the interim. For example, the federal district and circuit courts in the *Baby K* case (1994) relied on the Emergency Medical Treatment and Active Labor Act (EMTALA)[8] to order a continuation of artificial ventilation that was deemed futile or at least against standard medical practice by the health care providers involved.

---

[7] The abandonment argument has been used in two emerging issues in medical ethics: palliative care and assisted suicide. For example, some have called for greater use of palliative care for patients for whom life-sustaining treatments have been withheld or withdrawn: e.g., a physician's duty to care for his or her patient does not end with the cessation of aggressive life-support measures. Similarly, proponents of assisted suicide argue that physicians have a duty to provide the option of physician-assisted suicide to their terminally ill patients and that to withhold that option is tantamount to abandonment. Even further, some argue that if one accepts the legitimacy of physician-assisted suicide (and given the possibility that patients may be alone at the time of suicide and may botch the suicide attempt), "then the norm of nonabandonment supports physician presence at this moment" (Miller and Brody 1995:15).

[8] By enacting EMTALA, Congress created a positive right for indigent patients to receive emergency medical care – in effect, a right that compels doctors to touch patients for the purpose of providing medical care during an emergency regardless of their ability to pay for these services. However, it is unlikely that the Congress intended EMTALA to be used to resolve the futility problem.

Statutes addressing medical futility

To date, only a few statutes refer to futile or medically ineffective treatment. The types of statutes that embody the notion of futility include a federal act, DNR laws, and advance directive statutes governing living wills and medical powers of attorney. Some states go so far as to offer a method by which its citizens may request that all types of treatment be provided. Although it is unlikely that advance directive statutes would be interpreted as creating a positive right to receive any and all treatment, the legislatures that enacted these laws, as well as the individuals who rely on them, most likely believe they are protecting the patient's decision to be kept alive.

Federal legislation

Through the enactment of the Child Abuse Amendment Act in October 1984, Congress has already articulated a federal policy regarding futility. Although the provisions of the act apply only to neonates, its definition of futile treatment perhaps can be used to predict the language of any future federal legislation or regulation on the issue. The act may also provide support for a judicial finding of a right to receive treatment.

The Child Abuse Amendment Act ostensibly aims to protect handicapped infants from ''discriminatory'' behavior on the part of their parents or health care providers or both. This congressional intervention sought to end the controversy that erupted in 1982 when a minor surgical procedure was withheld from an infant born with Down syndrome. (See p. 51 for details about the Bloomington, Indiana, ''Infant Doe'' case and the futility debate concerning minors in general.) To combat the possibility of future discriminatory decisions, that is, decisions based on the likelihood of an infant surviving as a disabled person, the act requires all ''medically indicated treatment'' to be provided to neonates unless

(A) the infant is chronically and irreversibly comatose;
(B) the provision of such treatment would
   (i)   merely prolong dying,
   (ii) not be effective in ameliorating or correcting all of the infant's life-threatening conditions, or
   (iii) otherwise be futile in terms of the survival of the infant; or
(C) the provisions of such treatment would be virtually futile in terms of the survival of the infant and the treatment itself under such circumstances would be inhumane. (42 U.S.C. 5102(3))

By introducing "futile" twice into the section governing the withholding of medical treatment, Congress apparently expected to introduce reason into the debate about the care of severely handicapped neonates, acknowledging that some neonates suffering extreme distress will not survive even with the application of aggressive care.

In a 1989 report, the U.S. Commission on Civil Rights considered the Child Abuse Amendment Act. It noted that the futility exception to the mandate that requires physicians to treat critically ill neonates is a "cover all bases" approach that "ties futility to the 'survival' of the infant, emphasizing that only the inevitability of death despite treatment, and not the persistence of disability despite treatment, renders the treatment legally futile" (U.S. Commission on Civil Rights 1989:90). Thus, by defining futile treatment as a treatment that does not guarantee survival beyond the immediate crisis, the federal government applies a very narrow definition of futility to cases involving critically ill neonates.[9]

Interestingly, the first and only futility case to come before the federal judiciary (*Baby K* 1994) notably did not refer to the definition of futility in the Child Abuse Amendment Act. It is possible, however, that other federal courts may view the act as an indication of a broader federal policy regarding futility in future cases.

Do not resuscitate (DNR) legislation

One of the more recent trends in the refusal-of-treatment legislation is the enactment of DNR laws. (Currently 27 states have enacted do not resuscitate statutes.) A DNR order is a physician's written order not to attempt CPR on a particular patient. Although CPR was initially developed for unexpected cardiac and respiratory arrests following surgery or accidents, it is now commonly administered to anyone who arrests. It is presumed, unless otherwise indicated, that all patients would want to receive CPR.

Whereas every DNR law requires consent of either the patient or the surrogate before the order can be issued, a few statutes have adopted a futility

---

[9] According to the interpretative guidelines of the Department of Health and Human Services (DHHS), the third exception's requirement that the treatment be "virtually" futile, again in terms of survival, offers a lower threshold for a treatment to be considered futile. The guidelines interpret "virtually futile" to mean treatment that is "highly unlikely to prevent death in the near future" (45 C.F.R. pt. 1340 App. Interpretative Guideline §8 [1987]). However, the law conditions this reduced stringency on the requirement that the treatment also be "inhumane," an undefined qualifier that can be subjectively interpreted by different individuals and, therefore, offers little guidance.

rationale as a possible basis of withholding CPR in the absence of consent. That is, consent need not be secured to withhold a procedure that, in the opinion of the physician, should not be offered because it cannot benefit the patient.

Recent amendments to Georgia's DNR law may show a trend of introducing the concept of futility into the law. Before the amendment, the law stated (*Ga. Code Ann. §31-39-3[a]*)

Every patient shall be presumed to consent to the administration of cardiopulmonary resuscitation in the event of cardiac or respiratory arrest, unless there is consent or authorization for the issuance of an order not to resuscitate.

The 1994 Amendment added the following language to the same section: ''Such presumption of consent does not presume that every patient shall be administered cardiopulmonary resuscitation, but rather that every patient agrees to its administration unless it is medically futile.'' Medically futile is defined within the definition of ''candidate for nonresuscitation.'' A candidate in the original statute ''is a person for whom cardiopulmonary resuscitation would be medically futile in that such resuscitation will likely be unsuccessful in restoring cardiac and respiratory function or will only restore cardiac and respiratory function for a brief period of time so that the patient will likely experience repeated need for cardiopulmonary resuscitation over a short period of time.'' The 1994 amendment added, ''. . . or that such resuscitation would be otherwise medically futile.''

Tennessee regulations adopted in response to their DNR law have taken a similar approach. Under the rules promulgated by the Tennessee Department of Health, ''CPR may be withheld from the patient if in the judgment of the treating physician an attempt to resuscitate would be medically futile'' (Tenn. Hosp. Rules & Regulations §1200-8-4-.05[5][g]). Resuscitation efforts should be considered futile ''if they cannot be expected either to restore cardiac function to the patient or to achieve the expressed goals of the informed patient. In the case of the incompetent patient, the surrogate expresses the goals of the patient'' (Tenn. Hosp. Rules & Regulations § 1200–8–4–.05[3][h]).

New York also has adopted a law that allows physicians to write a DNR order for patients without capacity for whom there is no surrogate. The physician may issue the order, ''provided that the attending physician determines, in writing, that, to a reasonable degree of medical certainty, resuscitation would be medically futile . . .'' (N.Y. Pub. Health L. § 2966[1]). Medically futile is defined to mean that ''cardiopulmonary resuscitation will be unsuccessful in restoring cardiac and respiratory function or that the patient will experience repeated arrest in a short time period before death occurs" (N.Y. Pub. Health L. § 2961[12]).

Advance directive legislation

Two recently enacted advance directive statutes also address the futility issue. In 1995, both Maine and New Mexico enacted the Uniform Health-Care Decisions Act, a model law created by the National Conference of Commissioners on Uniform State Laws. The Maine act includes the following provision (Me. Rev. Stat. tit. 18-A, §5-807[f]).

A health-care provider or institution may decline to comply with an individual instruction or health-care decision that requires medically ineffective health care or health care contrary to generally accepted health-care standards.

The New Mexico version of the same model act adds the following statement to a section that is otherwise identical to Maine's: " 'Medically ineffective health care' means treatment that would not offer the patient any significant benefit" (N.M. Stat. Ann. § 24–7A-7[f]).

Other advance directive statutes use a similar approach by incorporating sections that would "protect" the physician from being forced to render treatment that is "medically inappropriate" (Louisiana), "medically ineffective" (Maryland), "medically unnecessary" (Virginia), "contrary to reasonable medical standards" (Oklahoma), or "not within accepted health care standards" (South Dakota).

At the other end of the spectrum, presumably in an attempt to create a semblance of neutrality, several living will statutes allow individuals to indicate what treatments they wish to receive, even if they become terminally ill, permanently unconscious, or otherwise critically ill without hope of recovery. Eleven living will laws[10] permit individuals to request life-sustaining treatment. Similarly, nine medical power of attorney statutes allow individuals to indicate their preference to receive medical care.[11]

The Indiana law goes as far as authorizing the use of a separate "Life Prolonging Procedures Declaration" as a final expression of one's "legal right to request medical and surgical treatment." (The option to request treatment in North Dakota's living will also includes similar language, explicitly

---

[10] Arizona, Idaho, Indiana, Kentucky, Maryland, Minnesota, North Dakota, Oregon, Pennsylvania, South Dakota, and Wisconsin.

[11] Georgia, Illinois, Kentucky, Maryland, Nevada, Oregon, Pennsylvania, South Carolina, and Vermont.

acknowledging a "legal right that medical or surgical treatment be provided.")

Three additional states[12] have distinct provisions for artificial nutrition and hydration in their living will laws, allowing individuals to reject all other life-sustaining treatments while simultaneously permitting them to indicate a desire to receive artificial nutrition and hydration. Even further, the Indiana law explicitly allows individuals to request artificial nutrition and hydration "even if the effort to sustain life is *futile* or excessively burdensome" (emphasis added).

The existence of statutes that permit patients to request life-sustaining treatment may or may not prove compelling to a court as establishing a state policy requiring physicians to provide treatment that they deem to be futile. In practice, the enactments of wrongful death and survivorship statutes over the years provide a powerful incentive within the medical profession to follow a family's request to treat a patient, even when the procedures involved generally would be considered futile by physicians and laypeople alike.

Judicial intervention in medical futility cases

The issue of futile treatment has been addressed on numerous occasions by the courts. However, until recently, the issue was approached from the perspective of a patient's right to refuse futile treatment being offered by a physician. Starting with *Quinlan*, numerous courts have relied on a determination that life-sustaining treatment was futile as one of the reasons for ordering the withholding or withdrawal of treatment.[13] Although these rulings relied primarily on the notion of the right to self-determination as the basis for their conclusions, the implication was that these decisions were especially appropriate because the treatments were considered futile.

The courts have only recently faced the prospect of deciding if an individual's wish to receive medical care should override a doctor's decision to

[12] Hawaii, Indiana, and Nevada.

[13] The New Jersey Supreme Court noted the following regarding Karen Ann Quinlan's wishes concerning life-sustaining treatment: "She was said to have firmly evinced her wish, in like circumstances, not to have her life prolonged by the otherwise futile use of extraordinary means" (*In re Quinlan* 1976:21). See also, *In re Dinnerstein* (1978:139) (". . . prolonged cardiac arrest dictates the futility of resuscitation efforts"); *Barber v. Superior Court* (1983: 491) (". . . there is no duty to continue its use once it has become futile in the opinion of qualified medical personnel"); *Bartling v. Glendale Adventist Medical Center* (1986:363) (". . . to provide continuous, but futile, life-sustaining treatment"); *In re Westchester County Medical Center* (1988:537) (". . . further treatment would not only be futile but painful"); *Westhart v. Mule* (1989:646) (". . . the effort will probably be futile and merely draw out the process of dying"); *In re Greenspan* (1989:1206) (". . . only when those measures would be futile"); *In re Lawrance* (1991:35) (". . . continued treatment is futile").

withhold or withdraw that care. Interestingly, each judicial intervention in a futility case, with one exception, has been in favor of continuing medical treatment, perhaps indicating the pervasiveness of the principle of patient autonomy. However, the lack of consistent reasoning in the decisions concerning the three significant cases to be discussed below is illustrative of the lack of consensus on the issue of medical futility within the law (Table 13.1).

The Wanglie *case*

The case that inaugurated the futility debate in recent years involved Mrs. Helga Wanglie, a patient at Hennepin County Medical Center (HCMC) in 1991 when a conflict developed between her family and her health care providers on the propriety of continuing mechanical ventilation (*In re Conservatorship of Wanglie* 1991). During the previous 18 months, Mrs. Wanglie had been shuffled between several health care facilities and suffered two cardiac arrests. Eventually, she was transferred back to HCMC, where her physicians suggested to Mrs. Wanglie's family a de-escalation of treatments, including the withdrawal of ventilator support. The family refused to consent to the withdrawal of mechanical ventilation, asserting that Mrs. Wanglie was a devout Lutheran and that her religious beliefs and those of her family precluded forgoing life-sustaining treatments. Arguing that Mrs. Wanglie's family and, in particular, her husband were not following the advice and counsel of her physicians, Dr. Steven Miles, a member of HCMC's ethics committee, petitioned the courts to replace Mr. Wanglie with a professional conservator as decision maker for Mrs. Wanglie. Finding no evidence that Mr. Wanglie could not make decisions for his wife, the court denied Dr. Miles' petition (*In re Conservatorship of Wanglie* 1991).

This case represented the first instance of a health care professional petitioning a court to order, albeit indirectly through the appointment of an ''impartial'' conservator, the cessation of life-sustaining care from an incompetent patient against the wishes of the patient's family. Because *Wanglie* was never appealed beyond the trial court level, it offers little precedential value to courts around the country. However, the value of this case is in the discussions it prompted across the nation about the limits of patient autonomy. In particular, it caused health, legal, and ethics professionals to reach a consensus that the issue of futility is no longer merely an academic issue or the meaningless ruminations of judges.[14]

---

[14] For example, in 1987, a Washington Court of Appeals noted the following regarding a claim for damages made by a patient and family against a health care provider who unilaterally

Table 13.1. *Court cases addressing futility*

The following cases address in some manner the issue of compelling a physician or health care facility to provide care to patients against the former's wishes or judgment. Although none of these cases is a typical futility case (as are *Wanglie*, *Baby K*, and *Gilgunn*), they may offer some precedential guidance to judges in future futility cases.

Alvarado v. N.Y.C. Health & Hospitals Corp., 145 Misc. 2d 687, 547 N.Y.S.2d 190 (Sup. Ct. N.Y. Co. 1989).
Health care providers were not obligated to provide life-support measures to brain dead patient despite the family's request for such treatment.

In re Jane Doe, 262 Ga. 389, 418 S.E.2d 3 (1992).
Statutory requirements prohibited the issuance of a DNR order unless both available parents consented. The Georgia Supreme Court also noted that because the minor patient's parents were in agreement that CPR should be provided, the trial court was correct to compel the hospital to provide CPR if Jane Doe suffered cardiac or respiratory arrest.

Dority v. Superior Court, 193 Cal. Rptr. 288 (1983).
Health care providers were not obligated to provide life-support measures to brain-dead patient despite the family's request for such treatment.

Kranson v. Valley Crest Nursing Home, 755 F.2d 46 (3d Cir. 1985).
A state-run nursing facility did not violate patient's constitutional rights by establishing a policy that instructs staff to withhold CPR from patients who suffer cardiac or respiratory arrest. (This policy can be mitigated by specifically requesting CPR in advance of any crisis.) The federal court also ruled that the facility's reliance on this policy and its decision to withhold CPR from a patient after he choked on a piece of meat did not constitute negligence and wrongful death.

Manning v. Twin Falls Clinic & Hosp., 830 P.2d 1185 (Ida. 1992).
Jury awarded compensatory and emotional distress damages against a hospital and nurse (and awarded punitive damages against only the nurse) for withdrawing oxygen support, despite family pleas, during room-to-room transfer that resulted in the patient's death. Although the family had consented to a DNR order, they alleged that the withdrawal of oxygen support caused the patient to suffer during the ordeal.

Moore v. Baker, 989 F.2d 1129 (11th Cir. 1993).
Physician was not required under consent statute to offer an alternative (to surgery) that is not "generally recognized and accepted by reasonably prudent physicians."

Payton v. Weaver, 182 Cal. Rptr. 225 (1982).
There is no legal obligation to provide care to an uncooperative and disruptive patient, even if patient competently requests the treatment. Also, hemodialysis treatment for chronic condition cannot be considered emergency care, and thus the laws that compel the provision of emergency care do not apply.

Table 13.1 (*cont.*)

Polikiff v. United States, 776 F. Supp. 1417 (S.D. Cal. 1991).
Veterans Administration hospital had no duty to provide AIDS testing for a patient and her spouse after it was determined that the patient had contracted hepatitis from her spouse. The court noted, ''there is no duty to provide a patient with information regarding a test when the testing is not recommended to the patient and would not be recommended to the patient by physicians of ordinary knowledge and skill.''

Strickland v. Deaconess Hosp., 735 P.2d 74 (Wash. App. 1987).
Patient and unrelated individuals' claims of damages were dismissed for various technical matters of law. The merits of the case were not decided. (Footnote 10 suggests that the court was sympathetic to the notion that health care providers should not unilaterally decide to withhold life-saving care.)

The Baby K *case*

A more recent case addressing the futility issue involved an anencephalic infant in Virginia, whose physicians petitioned a federal district court to withdraw ventilator care that had been provided since she was admitted to the hospital's emergency department for respiratory distress (*In re Baby K* 1994). The patient's mother insisted that the hospital was obligated to provide the care Baby K needed to continue living, despite a provision in the Virginia Health Care Decisions Act that explicitly permits physicians to withhold ''medically or ethically inappropriate'' health care. Relying on an expansive interpretation of EMTALA and the Americans with Disabilities Act, the district court agreed with Baby K's mother that treatment must be provided.

On appeal, the circuit court affirmed the decision but ruled only that EMTALA requires the provision of health care to every patient admitted in an emergency situation until the patient's emergency condition is stabilized. The court disagreed with the hospital's claim that Baby K's reason for admission through the emergency department was anencephaly, not respiratory distress. Instead, it noted that Baby K generally lived without ventilator support and was admitted to the hospital only when suffering respiratory distress. Therefore, the court argued that she was entitled to receive care until her

---

decided to withdraw ventilator support and issue a DNR order: ''Although the issue is ordinarily framed in terms of an individual's decision to *refuse* life sustaining treatment, we adhere to the fundamental common law and constitutional principles that 'competent adults have a right to determine what shall be done to their own bodies.' '' *Strickland v. Deaconess Hosp.* (1987) (citations omitted).

emergency respiratory problems were stabilized, even if these emergency admissions were based on a chronic condition. The circuit court further noted that the federal law precludes a state law from having effect if the two laws conflict, thereby making the provision of the Virginia Health Care Decisions Act inoperable in this situation. Importantly, the court did not review the substance of the hospital's contention – that ventilator care for anencephalic infants was futile and against prevailing medical standards.

In the *Wanglie* and *Baby K* cases, the judiciary has avoided discussing the merits of the futility argument, which is, ''Can a physician withhold or withdraw care that is deemed futile, or does a patient's right to autonomy require that futile care be provided?'' In both decisions, the courts ruled on narrow matters of law. Neither court ruled explicitly that individuals have the right to receive futile treatment.

The Gilgunn *case*

In *Gilgunn v. Massachusetts General Hospital*, a jury decided that the doctors were not negligent when they decided to withdraw mechanical ventilation and issue a DNR order despite the objection of the patient's daughter. The case was brought before the court after Mrs. Gilgunn's death. Mrs. Gilgunn's daughter also asked for damages for her own emotional distress in the case. In what was reported to be a two hour deliberation, the jury found that the hospital and doctors were not negligent in removing treatment from Mrs. Gilgunn despite their belief that she would have wanted to continue treatment. The decision was apparently based on the rationale that the treatment was futile (Kolata 1995). This case has been attacked by ethicists, who question the unilateral decision making of the attending physician (Capron 1995). It is interesting to note that the physician who was in charge of Mrs. Gilgunn's care before cessation of treatments revoked the DNR order after noting, ''I find it difficult to provide a medical reason to avoid CPR that is as powerful as their desire to have it done.''

This jury decision is the only court case to address the merits of the futility argument. It is also the only case that permitted health care providers to withhold and withdraw medical treatments against the patient's and family's wishes, although only retrospectively, based on the rationale that the treatment was futile.

Although *Gilgunn* is the most recent court decision to address medical futility, it would be premature to state that the tide has turned and that physicians are free to withhold or withdraw health care to patients on the basis of their belief that the treatment is futile. This case is unlike either *Wanglie* or *Baby K* not only because these rulings reached the opposite conclusion but also because the legal conflict in *Gilgunn* emerged only after the death of the patient. It is not unreasonable to speculate that a jury, or more likely, a judge might have ordered the continuation of treatment if presented with the case while Mrs. Gilgunn was still alive. Indeed, it is probably not difficult to convince someone – whether a judge or a lay jury member – that it is appropriate to continue treatment for a critically ill patient who is still alive because preventing the withdrawal of even futile treatment comes at little cost, whereas denying care is a violation of a living patient's desires and will result in the patient's death. It seems more difficult, however, to expect this same person to punish the physicians through a negligence lawsuit after the patient's death when presented with an argument that the treatments were futile and the physicians were making a medical decision in good faith. That is, the harm to an impersonal medical system in providing even futile care to the patient while alive is relatively minor, whereas the harm in punishing the physicians for stopping futile treatment may seem too drastic.

The three cases discussed and the nine cases listed in Table 13.1, demonstrate the lack of a legal consensus concerning medical futility. Moreover, these cases also illustrate the reluctance of the courts to definitively announce the limits, if any, of patient autonomy. Perhaps the courts prefer to have the issue resolved by society at large through the legislative process and the self-governance of health care professionals.

Conclusion

In essence, a futility case, like the refusal-of-treatment case, pits the patient's and family's desire for control over medical care against the physician's discretion in the practice of medicine. Meisel notes that the debate about futility cases, or what he calls "reverse" right-to-die cases, "is likely to occupy as much, if not more, judicial effort in the coming years as conventional right-to-die cases have in the last two decades unless legislation cuts it short" (Meisel 1995:530). Others doubt that this proliferation of cases will occur. Scofield, an outspoken advocate of the patient's right to refuse treatment, noted that, notwithstanding the volume of literature devoted to futility, "when patients are involved in decisions about medically futile treatment, they agree with their physician in more than 9 out of 10 cases" (Scofield 1994:67). He suggests that the futility problem can, in most instances, be preempted by encouraging an honest dialogue between doctors and patients.

There is undoubtedly at least a potential for an increase in the number of futility cases, especially in view of society's desire to curb the rising cost of health care. Although the courts may be able to address these conflicts on a case-by-case basis, such a scattershot approach will only invite further conflicts and litigation. The judiciary offers poor tools for reaching consensus. However, legislatures across the country may be better able to facilitate a consensus between medical professionals and health care consumers.

What is certainly needed, regardless of judicial and legislative activity, is a greater understanding among physicians and other health care providers that patients and families are often capable of rational discussion about their health care and that conflicts about whether to withdraw or to provide treatment can most likely be avoided by simply talking to patients. Similarly, patients and families must take greater responsibility and insist on becoming active participants in decisions concerning their care.

References

Capron A.M. 1995. Abandoning a waning life. *Hastings Center Report*. 24 (July–Aug):24–6.

Curtis, J.R., Park, D.R., Krone, M.R., and Pearlman, R.A. 1995. Use of the medical futility rationale in do-not-attempt-resuscitation orders. *Journal of the American Medical Association* 273:124–8.

Glick, H.R. 1992. *The Right to Die: Policy Innovation and Its Consequences*. New York: Columbia University Press.

Kolata, G. 1995. Court ruling limits rights of patients. *New York Times*. April 22, p. A6.

Kolata, G. 1994. Battle over a baby's future raises hard ethical issues. *New York Times*. December 27, p. A1.

Meisel, A. 1995. *The Right to Die*. New York: John Wiley & Sons, 2nd ed., vol. 2.

Miller, F.G., and Brody, H. 1995. Professional integrity and physician-assisted death. *Hastings Center Report*. 25 (May–June):8–17.

Mordarski, D.R. 1993. Medical futility: has ending life support become the next ''pro-choice/right to life'' debate? *Cleveland State Law Review* 41:751–87.

President's Commission for the Study of Ethical Problems in Medicine and Biomedical and Behavioral Research. 1983. *Deciding to Forego Life-Sustaining Treatment*. Washington, DC: Government Printing Office.

President's Commission for the Study of Ethical Problems in Medicine and Biomedical and Behavioral Research. 1981. *Defining Death*. Washington DC: Government Printing Office.

Scofield, G.R. 1994. Medical futility: can we talk? *Generations* Winter:66–70.

South Carolina Governor's Office, Division on Aging. 1994. *South Carolina State Survey*.

United States Commission on Civil Rights. 1989. *Medical Discrimination Against Children with Disabilities*.

Cases and statutes

In re Baby K, 16 F.3d 590 (4th Cir.), *cert. denied sub nom Baby K ex rel. Mr. K v. Ms. H*, 115 S. Ct. 91 (1994).

Barber v. Superior Court, 147 Cal. App. 3d 1006, 195 Cal. Rptr. 484 (Ct. App. 1983).

Bartling v. Glendale Adventist Medical Center, 184 Cal. App. 3d 961, 229 Cal. Rptr. 360 (Ct. App. 1986).

Child Abuse Amendments of 1984, 42 U.S.C. 5101 et seq.

Child Abuse Amendments of 1984 Final Rules, 45 C.F.R. pt. 1340 App. Interpretative Guideline § 8 (1987).

Chouinard v. Marjani, 575 A.2d 238 (Conn. Ct. App. 1990).

Cohen v. Smith, 648 N.E.2d 329 (Ill. App. 5 Dist. 1995).

Compassion in Dying v. Washington, 850 F. Supp. 1454 (D. Wash. 1994), *reversed*, 49 F.3d 586 (9th Cir. 1995).

Cruzan v. Director, Missouri Department of Health, 497 U.S. 261, 110 S. Ct. 2841 (1990).

In re Dinnerstein, 6 Mass. App. 466, 380 N.E.2d 134 (Ct. App. 1978).

Fox v. Smith, 594 So. 2d 596 (Miss. 1992).

Georgia act governing do-not-resuscitate orders, Ga. Code Ann. § 31-39-1 et seq.

Gilgunn v. Massachusetts General Hospital, No. 92-4820 (Mass. Super. Ct. Civ. Action Suffolk Co. April 22, 1995).

In re Greenspan, 137 Ill. 2d 1, 558 N.E.2d 1194 (1989).

Indiana Living Wills and Life Prolonging Procedures Act, Ind. Code Ann. § 16-8-4-11.

In re Lawrance, 579 N.E.2d 32 (Ind. 1991).

Leach v. Shapiro, 469 N.E.2d 1047 (Ohio Ct. App. 1984).

Louisiana Life-Sustaining Procedures Act, La. Rev. Stat. Ann. § 40:1299.58.1.

Maine Uniform Health-Care Decisions Act, Me. Rev. Stat. tit. 18-A, § 5-801 et seq.

Maryland Health Care Decision Act, Md. Health-Gen Code Ann. § 5-601.

Mohr v. Williams, 104 N.W. 12 (Minn. 1905).

New Mexico Uniform Health-Care Decisions Act, N.M. Stat. Ann. §§ 24-7A-1 et seq.

New York Orders Not to Resuscitate Act, N.Y. Pub. Health Law § 2961 et. seq.

New York Pub. Health L., § 2961 and 2966.

North Dakota Uniform Rights of the Terminally Ill Act, N.D. Cent. Code § 23-06.4-03.

Oklahoma Rights of the Terminally Ill or Persistently Unconscious Act, Okla. Stat. Ann. tit. 63, § 3101.12.

Perkins v. Lavin, 648 N.E. 839 (Ohio App. 9 Dist. 1994).

In re Quinlan, 70 N.J. 10, 355 A.2d 647, *cert. denied sub nom Garger v. New Jersey*, 429 U.S. 922 (1976).

Schloendorff v. Society of New York Hospital, 211 N.Y. 125, 105 N.E. 92 (1914).

Schmeltz v. Tracy, 177 A. 520 (Conn. 1935).

South Dakota Living Will Act, S.D. Codified Laws Ann. § 34-12D-19.

Strickland v. Deaconess Hosp., 735 P.2d 74 (Wash. App. 1987).

Tennessee regulations governing do-not-resuscitate orders, Tenn. Hosp. Rules & Regulations § 1200-8-4-.05.

Union Pacific R. Co. v. Botsford, 141 U.S. 250 (1891).

Virginia Health Care Decisions Act, Va. Code § 54.1-2990.

In re Conservatorship of Wanglie, No. PX-91-283 (Minn. Dist. Ct. Hennepin Co. July 1991).

In re Westchester County Medical Center, 72 N.Y.2d 517, 531 N.E.2d 607 (1988).

Westhart v. Mule, 213 Cal. App. 3d 542, 261 Cal. Rptr. 640 (Ct. App. 1989).

14

Professional and public community projects for developing medical futility guidelines

LINDA JOHNSON, M.S.W., AND
ROBERT LYMAN POTTER, M.D., PH.D.

Although exploration of medical futility usually begins with the professional community, the development of treatment abatement guidelines ought to consider the perspective of the public community as well. The professional and public communities must become partners in order to synthesize the two perspectives into a unified approach to the issue of medical futility. This synthesis is an example on the societal level of shared decision making between patient and physician on the clinical level.

This chapter describes specific attempts to develop futility guidelines for local public and professional communities, working separately and together. The projects were the topics of a meeting on the development of treatment abatement guidelines in situations of medical futility held in Kansas City, Missouri, January 26 and 27, 1996. The meeting was facilitated by the Midwest Bioethics Center, with generous funding from Employers Reinsurance Corporation and Hoechst Marion Roussel, Inc. Participants included project directors, national thought leaders, and Midwest Bioethics Center staff. A list of participants can be obtained from the authors.

Such shared decision making is one of the primary goals of the bioethics movement. Adequate attention to the diverse perspectives of differing moral communities when considering issues of respect for autonomy, beneficence, and justice will require careful compromise and search for a middle ground among multiple polarities. Consensus building in a morally pluralistic culture is a challenge to a liberal democratic society. Engelhardt's image of a "peaceable kingdom" achieved through negotiation among diverse moral communities is the organizing metaphor for this effort to develop treatment abatement guidelines in both the professional and public communities (Engelhardt 1996).

Professional community projects

Santa Monica, California

When Dr. Art Rivin, director of medical education, reviewed clinical cases with significant financial losses to the Santa Monica UCLA Medical Center, he became aware that one-third were patients transferred from nursing homes with acute illness superimposed on multiple chronic ailments or with severe dementia. The tremendous resources and intervention provided to these patients could not produce survival or restore a satisfactory quality of life. Out of this experience, the hospital developed a futile care policy through their bioethics committee and adopted it in early 1992. The policy defines futile care as any clinical circumstance in which the doctor and his consultants conclude from the available medical literature and their experience that further treatment other than comfort care cannot, within a reasonable possibility, cure, improve, or restore a quality of life that would be satisfactory to the patient.

Eighteen relevant cases have been reviewed by the bioethics committee since the adoption of the futile care policy. The information gained from these consultations, like the conclusions of the SUPPORT study (1995), provide information about where the problems develop in making decisions about appropriate end-of-life care.

The most common underlying problem was the attitude that death is the enemy and that because medicine is so advanced, a newly discovered technology might be effective in this case. Related to this was the fear of missing something and a compulsion to be thorough and complete and leave no possibility unexplored. Another concern was the doctor's excessive fear of a lawsuit. In some cases, the desire to please the family was the problem. In addition, a doctor who is on call or covering for a colleague is especially reluctant to withhold or withdraw care.

In most cases, adequate time and communication about the patient's goals and values, as well as realistic medical information, provided the basis for agreement. Conversations should begin early in the patient's hospitalization and must be gradual and realistic. However, those who believe that all life is precious and must be maintained, those who question the brain-death concept, and those who believe that a miracle will occur may never agree to comfort care only.

The Santa Monica project leaders concluded that the chief value of their policy on futile care is to raise awareness and communication among health care providers, patients, and families. They found that families as well as

physicians were sometimes unwilling to concede the futility of further intervention beyond comfort care. A multidisciplinary team conference is extremely useful but difficult to schedule and, therefore, often delayed.
Moreover, it is dependent on good communication and facilitation skills.
Other issues may influence the decision (e.g., age, self-inflicted injuries, social value) and must be carefully scrutinized. These same nonmedical issues
may also be a factor in populations who mistrust the medical community and
believe that they already receive insufficient care.

Participants in the Santa Monica project and in other projects described in
this chapter agreed on the need to include the public through education,
community meetings, and public policy initiatives in the process of evaluating
and decreasing the provision of futile care.

Minnesota project

This project, coordinated through the Minnesota Center for Health Care
Ethics by Dorothy Vawter, was developed to review current policies and
guidelines that address medical futility in Minnesota health care institutions.
The participants attempted to identify any emerging consensus within the
various policies that defined a community standard on futility and began by
identifying representatives of 38 health care institutions (36 hospitals, and 2
extended-care facilities) who were familiar with the end-of-life policies in
their institution. Two-thirds of the respondents were from ethics committees;
half were nurses.

The project concluded that there is nothing resembling a community standard on futility. Although 14 of the involved institutions have policies that
explicitly permit physicians to withhold or withdraw futile interventions, the
circumstances seen as relevant vary significantly. There was also great variability in the definitions of futility, standards required to justify a futility
judgment, procedural requirements and safeguards, and methods of resolving
conflicts.

There was consensus (87% of the institutional representatives) that model
futility guidelines would be useful to health care institutions in Minnesota.
Their first two goals, in rank order, would be to (1) protect patients from
useless and harmful interventions and (2) protect physicians and institutions
from legal exposure when they refuse to provide a futile intervention. Other
goals include protecting patients from mixed or confusing messages about
the possible efficacy of an intervention, unclear definitions of futility and lack
of benefit, and misapplied futility judgments and abuse.

The representatives also agreed to define a medically futile intervention as one (1) in which death is imminent and unavoidable or (2) that provides no benefit to the patient and is harmful as well. Procedurally, they agreed that a physician must obtain a second medical opinion confirming that the intervention would satisfy the definition of futility and that the physician should not be required to offer a patient a futile intervention but should be required to inform the patient/family when an intervention is futile and document the conclusion.

In regard to conflict resolution, the Minnesota group agreed that futility guidelines should offer guidance or requirements for resolving conflicts and that the advice of the ethics committee should be solicited. Also, they agreed that neither a patient/family's wishes nor a physician's judgment should always be the overriding factor. The group could not reach consensus on some issues, including funding: should a nonbeneficial, expensive treatment be considered futile if a patient/family is willing to pay for it?

This project is in its early stages, but the leaders are creatively developing an approach to prevent and resolve conflicts regarding futile interventions.

SUPPORT project

The SUPPORT project has been well reported in the medical literature (SUPPORT Principal Investigators 1995). As the recent article points out, even with attempts to integrate information and enhance communication in end-of-life decision making, impact and success were very limited. The study revealed many opportunities for improvement in communication, timing of decisions, and amelioration of pain. The authors also identified a need for improving the use of advance directives. Although illness and hospitalization had a significant impact on family resources (nearly one-third of the patients reported using up all or most of their savings), the authors concluded that instituting a strict prognosis-based futility standard would have only a moderate impact on societal health care costs.

The Center to Improve Care of the Dying, associated with the SUPPORT group, is initiating a project called MediCaring. Its goal is to develop and test the feasibility of a health care benefit that would enhance the provision of comprehensive supportive services to dying patients. The center is studying the potential to shift benefits for those at the end of life from hospital care to support care that emphasizes comfort, the patient's functional needs, and home care.

Houston, Texas, Citywide Task Force on Medical Futility

Twenty health care professionals, led by Baruch Brody, Ph.D., and Amir Halevy, M.D., have formed this citywide task force. It has brought together representatives from eight hospitals and one hospice and crossed disciplinary lines to create an alternative approach to processing the futility question (Baruch and Halevy 1995).

The initial controversial issues were (1) whether to define the term "futility" or replace it with "medical appropriateness" and (2) when and how inter-institutional and intra-institutional transfers should be handled. The group's work has gone through several draft stages and has now been distributed to all the participating institutions. Each institution is expected to develop its own policies in its institution-specific language and procedures while following the general outline of the guidelines. The Citywide Task Force will then draft legislation that reflects the content of the guidelines.

One of the recommendations of the task force was not to define futility; however, the guidelines do refer to treatments as medically inappropriate or medically futile. The third draft of the guidelines outlines a nine-step procedure that should be followed in evaluating the determination of futility. The procedure calls for dialogue between the attending physician and the patient or surrogate. Other options are also identified, including using chaplains or social workers, discussing possible transfer of care, and calling on the ethics committee. If these efforts fail to resolve any disagreement, an institutional review board can be called on to determine which clinical course should be followed. The goal of this process is to give a fair and equal hearing to patients and health care professionals while providing a mechanism for a final decision. These steps are not only checks; they are supports as well.

The draft guidelines were incomplete when they were presented at the Midwest Bioethics Center Seminar. However, community education on the concepts of the guidelines has begun. Since the guidelines were developed on a communitywide, professional basis, they offer the advantage that all who seek health care in Houston, from the indigent to the well insured, would function within the same guidelines. The untested questions are whether institutions will adopt policy based on the guidelines and whether physicians will invoke them.

Durham, North Carolina

Dr. Peter Kussin's participation in the SUPPORT study, combined with physicians' and the ethics committee's interest in having more helpful policies for end-of-life decision making led to a decision at Duke University Medical Center to try to develop medical futility guidelines. With significant institutional support and interest, they have developed and implemented policy and practice changes. Approximately two years ago, an initiative was started to take these conversations and developments to the entire state of North Carolina, under Dr. Kussin's direction.

Their goals were (1) to achieve broad representation of professional and community groups and (2) to maintain a neutral posture regarding the feasibility of developing community standards on medical futility. The diverse ideas of the panelists and speakers at a statewide conference were published (Sugarman 1995).

In North Carolina, the availability of excellent health care and deeply rooted individualistic notions of rights and freedoms make the public reluctant to discuss setting any limits on treatment. Managed care, which so far has little penetration in that particular health care market, is another untested variable.

The next phase in the North Carolina project will have two objectives: (1) professionals from all health care disciplines in which futility discussions are common will attempt to arrive at a consensus on what constitutes futile medical treatment, and (2) an effort will be made to achieve greater community participation in discussions about setting limits. Education and information will be essential, as will initiatives to develop more effective conflict resolution or mediation. To this end, 50 people have agreed to initiate conversations within local civic, cultural, religious, and other groups about setting health care limits at the end of life. These efforts will present opportunities not only to educate and inform the public but also to hear the groups' thoughts and ideas. In addition, a statewide organization has been established – the North Carolina Consortium to Set Limits in Medicine (NCCSLIM) – with representation from each of the diverse groups that were invited to the statewide conference. This consortium will be divided into regional working groups that will develop mission statements and an outline of objectives and activities.

Public community projects

Colorado Collective for Medical Decisions

Dr. Donald Murphy's Denver GUIDe project (now called the Colorado Collective for Medical Decisions, or CCMD) has been recognized as a primary example of a transitional type between professional and public community projects (Murphy and Barbour 1994). It started as heavily professional and has become more open to the public over the past three years.

The CCMD model has five committees working in the following areas: adult intensive care units, neonatal intensive care units, long-term care, legal issues, and public liaison. This report emphasizes the subcommittee on public liaison. It is made up of 20 health care professionals from hospitals and hospice programs and several members from the community; it meets monthly for an hour and a half.

Although the importance of involving the public was recognized early, the question of when to involve the public has been difficult to determine. Subcommittee members debated whether or not to include the broader community from the start, before any work had been done within the medical community, or to wait until the professional subcommittees developed recommendations regarding futile and inappropriate intensive care. The consensus was to lay the groundwork within the subcommittee and begin to develop guidelines before involving the public. The subcommittee established four goals: (1) to educate and be educated by the public, (2) to build consensus between CCMD and the public, (3) to establish a process that can be used again, and (4) to assist with research efforts.

The group has produced a 20-minute slide presentation with commentary that includes four case studies about futile care along with information about the goals of CCMD. Feedback from groups who have viewed the presentation are positive. An effort was made to include minority groups in the case studies.

A program of contacting churches, synagogues, and community groups has grown steadily, and an area hospital has published a brochure explaining the project. Through these contacts, more of the public has been involved in the discussion of these issues. A random telephone survey of 400 residents gathered important information about values, issues, and persons who will engage in the ongoing public dialogue. Both professional and public focus groups began in the fall of 1995, and town meetings are slated for 1996.

There has been some resistance from pro-life groups. The leadership of CCMD believes that it is important to engage diverse moral communities. They find it necessary to distinguish, in the public mind, their agenda from euthanasia and physician-assisted suicide. They believe that the Denver citizenry is ready to discuss difficult issues that the wider nation has not yet dealt with successfully.

The CCMD is successfully bridging the gap between the professional and public communities. How they work out this pathway will be instructive to other projects.

Sacramento, California: Extreme Care, Humane Options (ECHO)

The ECHO project, under Marge Ginsburg's leadership, is an interorganizational, interdisciplinary, community-wide, multiyear project to promote the provision of responsible, appropriate, and humane care for dying or irreversibly ill patients and their families. It covers the greater Sacramento region, which includes 14 acute care hospitals and 1.3 million people. Community guidelines will be created that integrate patient autonomy and responsibility, the knowledge of medical practitioners, and the values of an informed and diverse community.

Sacramento Healthcare Decisions (SHD), a nonprofit, nonpartisan community organization, sponsors and facilitates the project. Given the SHD purpose of educating and involving the public in health care policy and practice issues, the medical futility debate presented a valuable opportunity to address both sides of the issue: futile or inappropriate treatment being demanded by patients or families and inability or unwillingness of physicians to communicate clearly about palliative treatment options.

The temptation to address only one side of the issue (allowing physicians to refuse demands for inappropriate treatment) was strong, but to do so without facing the problem when patients and families are not making full use of their prerogative to refuse or demand treatment would be a disservice to all.

Having ascertained a strong interest among hospital bioethics committees to engage in an interorganizational effort, a steering committee was formed to develop the process, structure, and scope of ECHO. With SHD as the sponsor, it was clear that the public's role was not window dressing. Although the steering committee knew it wanted a workable process for arriving at mutually satisfactory patient–physician decisions, it could not predict whether the end results would include an Oregon-style list of things physicians did not have to do. With this understanding, a two-pronged process was begun: the public dialogue and the clinical dialogue.

The initial assumption was that the public needed to be educated so that it could understand the issue in the same way that health care providers do. However, it soon became clear that the purpose was to be educated by the public. With the use of case scenarios as discussion tools, the public dialogue (1) elicited the dominant (albeit often conflicting) values that underlie individual decisions about the use of technology for dying or irreversibly ill patients, (2) captured the hopes and fears that people expressed in considering the use of community guidelines, and (3) put into practice a seldom used concept of getting direct and explicit public input to create changes in health policy, not as a response to a finished product but before the guidelines were created.

This dialogue took place over a six-month period and involved more than 800 people in structured, interactive small group discussions of 8 to 12 people each. Fifty-two volunteer moderators were trained, and two moderators were used for each discussion, a discussion leader and a recorder. Although the process was highly qualitative, it produced a wealth of information about public concerns and values. It also generated a greater level of public interest and enthusiasm than anticipated. Although the intention was not necessarily to educate participants, it was clear that engaging in intense discussions about applying individual and societal values to dramatic medical dilemmas imparted new and thought-provoking knowledge.

Simultaneously, three interdisciplinary clinical committees were formed using Denver's model: adult intensive care, neonatology, and long-term care. Although the steering committee had concluded early that no attempt would be made to define futility, identifying specific indicators that put patients at risk for futile or inappropriate treatment was a goal of each clinical committee. Other aspects of providing care (e.g., improving communications, mechanisms for screening patients, a conflict resolution process) are also being discussed. The clinical committees will complete their work in 1996.

The Sacramento region has one of the highest concentrations of managed care in the country. Recent and often dramatic cost-cutting measures have made many local physicians hostile to anything that appears to reduce medical services. The cost issue is not presented as a driving force of ECHO, but some providers and consumers see for-profit HMOs lurking behind every change in health care practice. People are willing to save money by eliminating nonbeneficial treatment, but they do not want it to go to wealthy CEOs!

After additional input from the public and health care professionals (e.g., telephone survey, large community forum, review by hospital ethics committees, discussions with physician and hospital leadership), the final guidelines will be presented to the local hospitals for consideration and adoption. During the process, educational plans will be developed to ensure that the guidelines, in whatever form they are adopted, will not simply languish on the shelf.

Akron, Ohio

In 1994, an organizational meeting was attended by representatives from hospitals, physicians, extended care facilities, and local religious organizations in the Akron, Ohio, area. The purpose of the meeting was to develop a team approach to addressing several ethical issues regarding advance planning for medical decision making at the end of life. Steven Radwany, M.D., of Summa Health System and John Petrus, M.D., of the Akron General Medical Center convened this Collaborative Bioethics Working Group.

Over the next year, the group developed an identity, wrote a mission statement, and selected the name, Decisions, for the project. To maximize cooperation between the two hospitals in the area, the two physicians continued as cochairs of the project.

The mission statement sets the tone for the project.

To inform, prepare and empower physicians, health care providers, the public, and clergy to collaborate on difficult medical and bioethical issues, and to approach each unique situation with honesty, realism, sensitivity and regard for human dignity and autonomy.

The three areas of emphasis were education of the professions and the public, developing consensus on written guidelines, and the creation of a common language and unified forms to be used throughout the community.

The education committee would be responsible to

Develop community-wide educational activities or forums for physicians and other health care providers, patients, and families that help to create a greater awareness of death and dying issues, promote the use of advance directives, and address resource allocation in health care while helping to facilitate more open communication between patients and families and health care providers.

The guidelines committee would be responsible to

Develop care protocols, community standards, or guidelines, to be used when providing invasive, costly, high tech care at the margins of life. Develop a mechanism to encourage health care providers to anticipate and address such issues openly with patients and families.

The portability/common language development committee would be responsible to

Develop a dictionary of health care terminology and/or language that is acceptable community-wide. Develop a mechanism to improve the portability of DNR orders and other advance directives among all Summit County health care institutions (this may include the development of standard advance directive documents that could be used by all these institutions). If successful, the efforts of this group will help ease the difficulties families face when working with multiple caregivers at multiple institutions, and will ensure that the patient's wishes are better met.

A quarterly publication was planned for distribution to the professional and public communities. The main image of Decisions is that of "a community effort to help you make important health care decisions."

Recommendations about the use of cardiopulmonary resuscitation and percutaneous endoscopic gastrostomy tube placement have been tentatively developed but have not been widely adopted or presented to the public community. A common do not resuscitate (DNR) form has been created for the community.

This project was begun as a hospital-based and professional-based effort to achieve consensus within the health care community. Participation by the public community was not anticipated except to receive education regarding the guidelines. The leadership soon realized how important the use of public media could be for their project. A good relationship was nurtured with a health writer for a local newspaper, and a positive public image was created. The leaders have had useful meetings with groups of attorneys and clergy. Project leaders recognize the need for public input into the development of guidelines but have not yet created the structures through which to meet this need.

Appleton, Wisconsin

A conference sponsored by the Lawrence University Program in Biomedical Ethics, Network Health Systems, and United Health Group brought together faculty, resource persons, and health care professionals. Its goal was to determine whether a project could be designed to develop guidelines for the responsible use of intensive care. The participants emphatically concluded that such guidelines are needed. There was an equally strong consensus that the guidelines must not become legal mandates, nor should they be narrowly defined by futile care but should apply more broadly to inappropriate care. The conference recognized that the project must have input from an informed public from the outset and must be accompanied by an extensive education campaign for the general public. As a result, Wisconsin's project on Guidelines for the Responsible Utilization of Intensive Care (GRUIC) was set up, with Jack Stanley, professor of ethics and director of the Lawrence University Program in Biomedical Ethics at Lawrence University, Appleton, Wisconsin, as head.

Five working groups were established throughout Wisconsin in a pattern that followed the Denver project. Deliberations of the working groups focused on several major areas: (1) the definition of intensive care and its goals, (2) procedural methods that will help in establishing a balance between autonomy and paternalism, (3) the appropriateness or inappropriateness of legislation to support these guidelines, and (4) implementation of the guidelines.

The working groups confirmed the belief of the original conference participants that the guidelines should not be created with the goal of a legislative mandate. However, since legislation may be a secondary result of the guidelines, painstaking care must be taken in their creation. The primary goal is to create guidelines rooted in practice, as well as literature to guide responsible decision making for all parties in situations involving intensive care. The neonatal intensive care group had particular concerns about legislation in the wake of the federal Baby Doe regulations, which left many in the neonatology field more confused than enlightened.

The second phase of the project began in March, 1996, when the guidelines were brought to three kinds of discussion groups across the state: groups of the general public, health care professionals, and other professionals. The public groups will have open meetings based on the Georgia Health Decisions Model. They will read and discuss drafts of the guidelines and prepare critical responses to be considered by the five original working groups before the guidelines are finalized. The two professional groups will also read, discuss, and critique the guidelines, as will selected individual readers who are not group members. For the preparation of the general public discussion groups, project leaders are working on an educational design to be funded by the Wisconsin Humanities Council. This series of forums throughout the state will prepare the public to respond to the drafts, which will be informed by accurate information and examined public values. The educational dimension of the project will be carried out by Wisconsin Health Decisions in cooperation with the Lawrence University Program in Biomedical Ethics.

Other projects

The American Medical Association (AMA) was represented at the Midwest Bioethics Center's meeting by John Crosby, J.D., who is supervising the AMA committee charged with developing various clinical guidelines. All project leaders recognized the importance of coordinating various health care professional societies in developing statements and procedures. It is not necessary that complete unanimity be achieved, but dialogue and understanding of differing positions are required to move the development and acceptance of guidelines. The AMA represents a collaborative attitude that is shared by many other professional societies. This cooperative spirit will be useful for guiding other communities that may be interested in developing their own guideline projects.

References

Baruch, A.B., and Halevy, A. 1995. The role of futility in health care reform. In *Health Care Crisis? The Search for Answers*. Misbin, R.I., Jennings, B., Orentlicher, D., and Dewar, M., eds., pp. 31–40. Frederick, MD: University Publishing Group.

Engelhardt, H.T., Jr. 1996. *Foundations of Bioethics*, 2nd. ed. New York: Oxford University Press.

Murphy, D.J., and E. Barbour. 1994. GUIDe (Guidelines for the Use of Intensive Care in Denver): a community effort to define futile and inappropriate care. *New Horizons* 2:326–31.

Sugarman, J., ed. 1995. Issue on perspectives on medical futility. *North Carolina Medical Journal* 56, No. 9.

The SUPPORT Principal Investigators. 1995. A controlled trial to improve care for seriously ill hospitalized patients. The Study to Understand Prognoses and Preferences for Outcomes and Risks of Treatments (SUPPORT). *Journal of the American Medical Association* 274:1591–8.

15

Community futility policies: the illusion of consensus?

BETHANY SPIELMAN, PH.D, J.D.

The longer the problem of medical futility persists, the smaller will be the percentage of difficult futility cases that are resolved entirely between physicians and patients or their surrogates. Like many medical ethics problems, futility has become a matter of institutional, legislative, judicial, and scholarly concern. This is not unusual. What is unusual is the degree to which the issue of futility has been identified as a matter of community concern. For example, a brochure advertising a recent conference titled ''A Community Policy on Medical Futility?'' included the statement, ''We believe that implementation of a consensus community standard embracing the full spectrum of public and professional opinion is the only way to ensure rational and ethical guidelines for medical practice'' (Duke University 1995). Efforts across the country to develop community futility policies are underway in Colorado, California, Texas, and elsewhere (see Chapter 14).

For example, a citywide task force on medical futility has been established in Houston. Professionals from nine health care organizations are participating. After a basic philosophy was agreed on, a committee began to develop guidelines to help member institutions develop institutional futility policies and to draft and obtain support for legislation consistent with those guidelines. The committee produced four principles and nine procedural steps, which have been summarized by Pentz (Pentz 1995)

GUIDe (now called The Colorado Collective for Medical Decisions) is a group of Denver health care providers that began organizing in 1993 to create community clinical standards for withholding futile treatment. Five task forces were established: adult intensive care, long-term care, neonatal intensive care, public education and liaison activities, and a legal task force. The plan for the project has been to build consensus about recommendations generated by the three medical task forces among GUIDe members and then obtain feedback from the larger medical community. GUIDe plans to involve the public through religious and civic organizations and public survey instruments (Buchanan 1995; Using SUPPORT to GUIDe 1995).

This chapter, which reflects some skepticism about community futility policies (although not about all futility-related community projects) identifies factors that seem to drive these efforts. Then, it evaluates the uses to which community futility policies might be put. I suggest that although health care organizations need futility policies and could make use of the additional data that cooperative research projects on futility policies might generate, the hope that community efforts to develop futility policies will generate better definitions of futility or fundamentally new procedures for handling futility cases is misguided.

What drives community efforts to develop futility policies?

The turn to community projects as a solution to futility problems has been driven by several beliefs and concerns. First, community efforts are consistent with the widespread belief that futility is a problem of distributive justice that society should have a voice in resolving. Because the costs of futile medical interventions are not borne by patients and families alone, advocates of community polices believe that society, or "the community," should have a voice in decisions about futile treatment. Some commentators have argued that the cost problem and the futility problem are linked so closely that they cannot be understood separately. For this group, social costs – to society in general, or to a particular group of insurance subscribers – dictate community solutions; cost and futility are a single problem (Murphy and Finucane 1993). Other commentators, however, insist on distinguishing the issues (Jecker and Schneiderman 1992; Tomlinson and Czlonka 1995).

Second, after the Helga Wanglie case (*In re Conservatorship of Wanglie* 1991) and particularly after the Baby K decision (*In the Matter of Baby K* 1994), health professionals began to recognize that courts will not always defer to physician judgments about futility and will sometimes frame the futility problem in ways that are quite different from what health care providers expect. Disappointed with these legal results, those involved in developing futility policies may hope that other entities than courts will become the final arbiters of futility. This could happen if health care professionals were able to persuade patients and families to stop demanding treatment because it is inconsistent with community values or if physicians were emboldened to withhold futile treatment because of evidence that their beliefs about futility were widely held. Resorting to courts could also be avoided if health care professionals could invoke, in the clinical setting, a statute enacted with the political support of health care facilities (Spielman 1994a, 1995, Pentz 1995).

Third, if a malpractice suit arose out of a futility dispute, evidence about the standard of care would be presented in court. This evidence, in the form of expert testimony, would be necessary for a jury to determine whether a physician had a duty to provide the disputed treatment or a duty to take certain procedural steps before discontinuing it. Advocates of community policies also believe it would be helpful to articulate a standard of care in advance of such a lawsuit. Under the right conditions, community futility policies could thus serve as a new source of evidence for the defense in medical malpractice suits (Buchanan 1995).

Fourth, communitarian ethics is in vogue. The last 10 years have seen a dramatic increase in appeals to the public good rather than to individual rights as sources of ethical guidance and to communitarianism rather than individualism as the paradigm of moral thinking. A communitarian approach to problems has widespread appeal, and the communitarian literature in medical ethics is growing (Sandel 1982; Emanuel 1991; Brody 1993; Etzioni 1993; Callahan 1994; Zoloth-Dorfman 1995). At a time when a return to community is viewed as a solution to so many of the ills of modern society, it is not surprising that community approaches also attract those interested in resolving futility problems.

Finally, some may hope that a communitarian approach could moderate the tension between patient autonomy and physician autonomy. If communities that include both physicians and patients can develop ways to resolve futility conflicts, their resolutions might be viewed as less divisive and more authoritative than resolutions emanating from health care professionals alone or from patients alone. The community might function, under the right circumstances, as a kind of neutral arbitrator.

Proposed goals for community efforts

Defining futility

Whether community futility policies are ultimately found to be worth the effort required to develop them depends, in part, on what they are intended to accomplish. I suggest that it is unlikely that these projects will generate better or even different answers than others have already produced by other means.

Some community efforts are expected to answer the substantive question "What should count as futile treatment?" The GUIDe project in Denver is developing what its leaders hope will become a community policy incorporating very specific criteria for determining futility. One of its task forces has recommended, for example, that aggressive life support be forgone for infants with trisomy 13 or 18, Potter's disease, or anencephaly. Another has suggested that transfer to an ICU is futile for patients in a persistent vegetative state (Buchanan 1995).

As Tomlinson and Czlonka have pointed out, however, defining futility, whether by setting quantitative standards or by identifying categories of patients who should not be treated, creates several risks. Defining futility creates the illusion of specificity where none is possible; it may lead to superficial medical evaluations, and it ties futility to narrow biomedical goals for the patient (Tomlinson and Czlonka 1995).

Many approaches to the subject of futility found in the literature, institutional policies, and the law are problematic from this perspective. Some go farther than others toward "creating the illusion of specificity." For example, Schneiderman, Jecker, and Jonsen (1990) have defined a treatment as futile if "physicians conclude (either through personal experience, experiences shared with colleagues or consideration of reported empirical data) that in the last 100 cases, a medical treatment has been useless." A futility policy used by the Johns Hopkins Hospital states: "Any course of treatment may be regarded as futile if it is highly unlikely to have a beneficial outcome, or it is highly likely merely to preserve permanent unconsciousness or persistent vegetative state or require permanent hospitalization in an intensive care unit . . ." (Johns Hopkins 1992; Waisel and Truog 1995). New York's do not resuscitate (DNR) law defines medically futile CPR as "cardiopulmonary resuscitation [that] will be unsuccessful in restoring cardiac and respiratory function or that [will result in] the patient . . . experience[ing] repeated arrests in a short time period before death occurs" (N.Y. C.L.S. Pub. Health L. 2961 1991). From Tomlinson and Czlonka's perspective, this whole family of futility definitions, whether generated by community-wide efforts, legislatures, health care facilities, or scholars, is misbegotten.

Community policies present additional problems. If they are to carry moral weight, collective judgments about which lives are worth extending and which are not should be built on processes that are open to divergent points of view (Caws 1991; Jennings 1991; Moreno 1995). Without openness to potential dissenters and conscientious objectors, community efforts could degenerate into forced consensus (Spielman 1994b; Post 1995). Unfortunately, the idea of community has not coexisted easily with cultural, ethnic, and religious pluralism (Phillips 1993). Although many in society currently long for community and the consensus it implies, agreement about values does

not exist even in relatively homogeneous groups, such as physicians or residents of a narrow geographic area. Suppression of divergent beliefs and
value systems hardly seems desirable because some futility disputes arise
from fundamental differences in worldviews.

The Ryan Nguyen (or *Baby Ryan*) case illustrates the kind of case in which
both family and physicians acted on minority views about the definition of
futility. Ryan Nguyen was born prematurely, with an intestinal blockage,
possible brain damage, and kidney failure at Sacred Heart Medical Center in
Spokane, Washington, in late 1994. After Sacred Heart physicians recommended, on the basis of their notion of futility, that Ryan's life support be
withdrawn, the infant's parents obtained a court order to force the hospital
to continue treatment. The Nguyens did not view the treatment as futile.
Physicians at Legacy Emanuel Hospital in Portland, Oregon, thought the
treatment would not be futile and agreed to provide it. Ryan was treated and
discharged home in March of 1995 and was not expected to need a kidney
transplant as an infant (Capron 1995; Glamser 1995; Kolata 1995; J. Cox,
personal communication, May 10, 1995).

Many physicians – perhaps most – would have labeled the disputed treatment futile and decided to forgo life-sustaining treatment in the Nguyen case.
Many parents – perhaps most – would have labeled the treatment futile and
wanted to forgo treatment for their infant. My point is not simply that because
the infant survived, these minority views about what counts as futile treatment
were right and the majority wrong. Rather, these minority viewpoints were
"right enough" that a community futility project could not justifiably discount or dismiss them. Health care professionals cannot ignore existing differences in religions, cultures, and medical practice styles if they wish to do
their jobs well, yet it is precisely those differences that proponents of community policies may have to gloss over, suppress, or label as "special interests" in the quest for a one-size-fits-all definition of futility.

Prescribing procedures

Community efforts are also addressing the procedural question, "What
should be done when treatment desired by the patient or family is thought
by the physician to be futile?" The phenomenon of community efforts suggests that the usual resources, that is, institutional ethics committees, consultants, scholarly efforts, and legislative and judicial processes, are
inadequate to resolve futility problems. Legislative processes, courts, or ethics
committees and consultants are all vulnerable to criticism, yet they seem to

have generated a menu of options for physicians that will not change significantly once community policies have been developed.

What approaches have been produced? Physicians can, of course, take any number of steps to ensure that disagreements do not harden into irreconcilable disputes (West and Gibson 1992; Dubler and Marcus 1994), but when disputes do harden, five basic approaches have emerged through ethics committee, legislative, and scholarly processes.

First, a physician can, with the concurrence of colleagues or an ethics committee or both, decide to stop treatment. For example, in 1989, physicians at Massachusetts General Hospital decided to end treatment for Catherine Gilgunn. The 71-year-old patient, who suffered irreversible neurologic damage and multiple system failure following a hip fracture, had wanted to have everything done to sustain her life, according to her daughter, Joan Gilgunn. After consultation with the chair of the hospital's optimal care committee, physicians issued a DNR order and began to wean the patient off ventilator support over her daughter's objections. Catherine Gilgunn died shortly thereafter ("To treat or not to treat" 1995; Kolata 1995).

A similar approach was used in a case involving a young child on extracorporeal membrane oxygenation, described by Paris et al. (1993). Likewise, Veterans Affairs Hospitals are governed by a policy that permits discontinuation of treatment over family requests (Veterans Health Administration 1993; Sadler and Mayo 1993).

In the second approach, with the cooperation of the hospital's attorney, a physician can continue treatment and commence legal action. This occurred in the *Wanglie* case, when physicians continued ventilator support while Hennepin County Medical Center filed a petition requesting that an independent third party be appointed as decision maker. This approach was also used in the *Baby Ryan* case, although the legal action involved was highly questionable. Health professionals at Sacred Heart Medical Center filed a child abuse complaint against the infant's parents for insisting on treatment physicians believed futile. The child abuse complaint was dropped when the infant was transferred to another hospital (Kolata 1994; Capron 1995; Glamser 1995).

Third, a physician can continue treatment until the patient is transferred. This approach is required by Minnesota and Virginia statutes. The Virginia Health Care Decisions Act states (Va. Code Ann. 1994)

An attending physician who refuses to comply with the advance directive of a qualified patient or the treatment decision of a person designated to make the decision (i) by the declarant in his advance directive or (11) pursuant to sec.54.1-2986 shall make a reasonable effort to transfer the patient to another physician. This section shall apply even if the attending physician determines the treatment requested to be medically or ethically inappropriate.

The Minnesota statute states the approach even more clearly (Minn. Stat. 1994).

A health care provider who is unwilling to provide directed health care under paragraph (a) that the provider has the legal and actual capability of providing may transfer the principal or declarant to another health care provider willing to provide the directed health care but the provider shall take all reasonable steps to ensure provision of the directed health care until the principal or declarant is transferred.

Of course, these and other legal requirements to facilitate or permit patient transfers limit the potential of community futility policies to create what some developers want to create, a uniform standard of care. The standard of care would be described differently by the physicians from whom patients have received the disputed intervention and by the physicians who prefer to transfer the patient rather than provide the disputed intervention. Even in states that do not statutorily require transfers, health care professionals at the facility in which a patient initially receives care cannot legally block a transfer to another facility that is willing to provide the disputed intervention (Zupanec 1994). If finances are not an obstacle, a community policy cannot prevent the patient from obtaining the treatment when another health care facility is willing to provide it.

The case of the Lakeburg twins, who were joined at the chest and shared a heart, illustrates that the transfer option has been used in futility cases since 1993. The twins were born to Kenneth and Reitha Lakeburg in Illinois in 1993. Physicians at Loyola University Medical Center refused to perform surgery to separate the twins because they estimated the chance of even one surviving at only 1%. The twins were transferred to Children's Hospital of Pennsylvania, however, where the girls' single heart was restructured so that one of the infants would have a chance to survive (Rosenthal 1993).

Fourth, physicians can continue treatment until the patient's medical condition changes. This approach was used, apparently by default and with some frustration, in a case described by Koch, Meyers, and Sandroni (1992). A 45-year-old minister who experienced cardiac arrest on a dialysis unit developed cerebral edema and became comatose. His family contacted the police and media and accused one of the attending critical care physicians of being possessed by the devil. The hospital attempted to call in an outside consultant, held meetings with the medical center president, chief of staff, and legal counsel, and considered going to court. In the end, the patient received dialysis until he was pronounced brain dead (Koch et al. 1992).

Finally, physicians in some geographic areas can ask for review by an expert panel as an alternative to judicial review. In Denver, a nonjudicial model of case review for allegedly futile treatment is being developed as a pilot program by several universities (Buchanan 1995). Panel review in this model is a mandatory precursor to judicial appeal and could prevent litigation of some futility cases. This approach resembles prelitigation screening panels, established as a form of alternative dispute resolution in several jurisdictions across the country (Begel, 1995).

These five approaches seem to me to be a comprehensive list of options that will not be significantly expanded by further community efforts. The facts of some cases will require minor modifications of these choices, but these five approaches will likely exhaust the basic options for resolving futility disputes. If community policies are expected to generate new options for the most difficult cases, it is unlikely that developers' expectations will be met.

More appropriate goals for community efforts

Although some community efforts to establish policies for futility decisions are questionable, others could be quite worthwhile. Under the right circumstances, community futility policies could contribute to our understanding of the kind of futility policies that work best. If several health care facilities reached an agreement about what might be an effective policy and pooled their resources so that the policy could be rigorously evaluated, they would generate more useful data than a single facility that established and evaluated the same policy. Empirical studies that assess the effectiveness of ethics-related hospital policies are virtually nonexistent in the clinical ethics literature. A community effort directed toward such an inquiry might eventually make an important contribution toward solving futility disputes in more constructive ways.

There are, of course, many good reasons for developing single-organization futility policies (Stell 1992). Health care organizations are the places in which medical decisions are made, medical interventions are provided, and ethics consultations are carried out. They are the entities that risk legal liability when disputes are handled poorly. Providers within those institutions need to know what resources are available to them for resolving futility disagreements, what steps they should take if disagreements harden into disputes, and why. Institutions need to decide whether to proceed in ways that either encourage prevention of futility conflicts, minimize cost, or minimize legal risk. They also need to decide when to initiate or accept transfers of patients involved in futility disagreements, and they must clearly communicate those conditions to patients and families. Often, institutions are responsible for teaching students and residents how to deal with medical ethics problems. A futility policy can help with each of these tasks.

Conclusion

I have suggested that some community efforts that focus on futility policies are potentially more problematic than others. The primary goal of community efforts should not be to generate new substantive or procedural approaches to futility problems. Community efforts can add little to what individual health care organizations are already learning and doing to resolve futility issues. Efforts focused on these goals are unlikely to produce enough of significance to justify devoting additional community resources to the scholarly, institutional, legislative, and judicial resources already expended on this problem. However, if the primary goal is to learn which policies work well and which do not, community efforts might eventually contribute significantly to resolving these problematic situations.

References

Begel, J. 1995. Maine physician practice guidelines: implications for medical malpractice litigation. *Maine Law Review* 47:69–103.

Brody, B.A. 1993. Liberalism, communitarianism and medical ethics. *Law and Social Inquiry* 2:393–408.

Buchanan, S.F. 1995. What constitutes futile treatment and guidelines? In *Health Care Crisis? The Search for Answers*, Misbin, R.I., Jennings, B., Orentlicher, D., and Dewar, M., eds., pp. 49–59. Frederick, MD: University Publishing Group.

Callahan, D. 1994. Bioethics: private choice and common good. *Hastings Center Report* 24 (May–June):28–31.

Capron, A.M. 1995. Baby Ryan and virtual futility. *Hastings Center Report* 25(March–April):20–1.

Caws, P. 1991. Committees and consensus: how many heads are better than one? *Journal of Medicine and Philosophy* 16:375–91.

Dubler, N.N., and Marcus, L.J. 1994. *Mediating Bioethical Disputes. A Practical Guide*, New York: United Hospital Fund of New York.

Duke University Medical Center Ethics Committee and the Office of Continuing Medical Education. 1995. A community policy on medical futility? A conversation of the North Carolina community, March 10. Durham, NC: Duke University.

Emanuel, E. 1991. *The Ends of Human Life: Medical Ethics in a Liberal Polity.* Cambridge, MA: Harvard University Press.

Etzioni, A. 1993. *The Spirit of Community: Rights, Responsibilities and the Communitarian Agenda.* New York: Crown Publishers.

Glamser, D. 1995. "Miracle Baby" puts new life in ethics debate. *USA Today*, January 16, p. A7.

Jecker, N.S., and Schneiderman, L.J. 1992. Futility and rationing. *American Journal of Medicine* 92:189–96.

Jennings, B. 1991. Possibilities of consensus: toward democratic moral discourse. *Journal of Medicine and Philosophy* 16:447–63.

Johns Hopkins Hospital, 1992. *The Johns Hopkins Hospital Policy on Withholding or Withdrawing Futile Life-Sustaining Medical Interventions*. Baltimore, MD: Johns Hopkins Hospital.

Koch, K.A., Meyers, B.W., and Sandroni, S. 1992. Analysis of power in medical decision-making: an argument for physician autonomy. *Law, Medicine and Health Care* 20:320–9.

Kolata, G. 1994. Battle over a baby's future raises hard ethical issues. *New York Times*, December 27, p. A1.

Kolata, G. 1995. Court ruling limits rights of patients. *New York Times*, April 22, sec. 1, p. 6.

Moreno, J. 1995. *Deciding Together: Bioethics and Moral Consensus*. New York and Oxford: Oxford University Press.

Murphy, D.J., and Finucane, T.E. 1993. New do-not-resuscitate policies: a first step in cost control. *Archives of Internal Medicine* 153:1641–8.

Paris, J.J., Schreiber, M.D., Statter, M., et al. 1993. Beyond autonomy – physicians' refusal to use life-prolonging extracorporeal membrane oxygenation. *New England Journal of Medicine* 329:354–7.

Pentz, D. 1995. The need for a community-wide futility policy: or, how not to handle a case of medical futility. In *Health Care Crisis? The Search for Answers*. Misbin, R.I., Jennings, B., Orentlicher, D., and Dewar, M. eds. pp. 41–8. Frederick, MD:University Publishing Group.

Phillips, D. 1993. *Looking Backward:A Critical Appraisal of Communitarian Thought*. Princeton, NJ:Princeton University Press.

Post, S.G. 1995. Baby K: medical futility and the free exercise of religion. *Journal of Law, Medicine & Ethics* 23:20–6.

Rosenthal, E. 1993. One Siamese twin survives an extraordinary separation. *New York Times*, August 21, sec. 1, p. 1.

Sadler, J., and Mayo, T. 1993. The Parkland approach to demands for "futile" treatment. *HEC Forum* 5(1):35–8.

Sandel, M. 1982. *Liberalism and the Limits of Justice*. Cambridge: Cambridge University Press.

Schneiderman, L.J., Jecker, N.S., and Jonsen, A.R. 1990. Medical futility: its meaning and ethical implications. *Annals of Internal Medicine* 112:949–54.

Spielman, B. 1994a. Collective decisions about medical futility. *Journal of Law, Medicine & Ethics* 22:152–60

Spielman, B. 1994b. Futility and conscience. Paper presented at the 22nd Annual Meeting on Value Inquiry, Drew University, Madison, NJ, April 21–23.

Spielman, B. 1995. Bargaining about futility. *Journal of Law, Medicine & Ethics* 23:136–42.

Stell, L. 1992. Stopping treatment on grounds of futility: a role for institutional policy. *Saint Louis University Public Law Review* 11:481–97.

To treat or not to treat: a closer look at unilateral decisions. 1995. *Hospital Ethics* 11(3):6–8.

Tomlinson, T., and Czlonka, D. 1995. Futility and hospital policy. *Hastings Center Report* 25 (May–June):28–35.

Using SUPPORT to GUIDe our fix on futility. 1995. *Hospital Ethics* 11(1):2–5.

Veterans Health Administration, Department of Veterans Affairs. 1993. Withholding and withdrawal of life-sustaining treatment. In *Manual M-2, Clinical Affairs, Part I. General.* Washington, DC: Department of Veterans Affairs.

Waisel, D.B., and Truog, R.D. 1995. The cardiopulmonary resuscitation-not-indicated order: futility revisited. *Annals of Internal Medicine* 122:304–8.

West, M., and Gibson, J. 1992. Facilitating medical ethics case review: what ethics committees can learn from mediation and facilitation techniques. *Cambridge Quarterly of Healthcare Ethics* 1:63–74.

Zoloth-Dorfman, L. 1995. Community and conscience. In *Health Care Crisis? The Search for Answers*, Misbin, R.I., Jennings, B., Orentlicher, D., and Dewar, M., eds., pp. 223–34. Frederick, MD: University Publishing Group.

Zupanec, D. 1994. False imprisonment in connection with confinement in nursing home or hospital. *American Law Reports* 4:449.

Cases and statutes

In re Conservatorship of Wanglie, No. PX-91–283 (Minn. Dist. Ct. Hennepin Co. July 1991).

In the Matter of Baby K, 16 F.3d 590 (4th Cir.), *cert. denied*, 115 S.Ct. 91 (1994).

Minn. Stat. § 145C.15 (1994).

N.Y.C.L. Pub. Health L. 2961 (1991).

Va. Code Ann. § 54.1–2987 (1994).

16

Not quite the last word: scenarios and solutions

KAREN ORLOFF KAPLAN, M.P.H., SC.D.

In 1995, the editors of this book asked a group of outstanding scholars and clinicians to consider the concept of medical futility with 1995 eyes – to discuss current understanding, practices, and concerns about this complex, emotionally fraught, multifaceted subject. This is a timely consideration because reaching consensus about medical futility paradigms and consistently applying them has become increasingly challenging. The health care system's exploding technologic capacity, soaring health care costs, greater focus on end-of-life treatment decisions, and expanding concerns about blending health care consumer empowerment with community needs are making the futility debate more and more contentious.

In his well-considered summary of a 1993 professional meeting dedicated to the question of medical futility, Pearlman (1994) raises a threshold question. "Why," he asks, "has medical futility become a battleground between physicians and patients (or their family members), rather than an area for thoughtful deliberation and negotiation?" The answer, or rather answers, to Pearlman's question lie in the pivotal concepts and concerns articulated at the meeting that he summarized (Fins 1994) and in the present volume. These publications discuss the most likely future scenarios for our nation's approach to the question of medical futility.

Summary of preceding chapters

Because the concept of medical futility and models for its application are so complex and the subject is so emotionally laden, many experts question the usefulness of the concept. Some consider its unilateral application, that is, that the physician makes the decision, a particularly dangerous overstepping of the physician's role and an assault on patient autonomy. Howard Brody (Chapter 1) reviews the arguments against the concept of medical futility,

179

noting primarily that there is no consensus about its definition or about guide-lines for making futility judgments. In too many instances, we lack the sci-entific data needed to determine the efficacy of a treatment and, therefore, risk mistaking judgments based on physicians' values for fact-based deci-sions.

However, Brody stresses that the concept of medical futility cannot be disregarded entirely. Indeed, he suggests that in view of the realities of med-ical practice and the need to preserve physicians' professional integrity, there is no way to avoid futility judgments in practice. He discusses situations in which even a unilateral physician decision to withhold treatment seems jus-tified, for example, when the treatment has no pathophysiologic rationale, the patient is not responding regardless of dose, or the treatment already has been tried unsuccessfully or has no reasonable chance of meeting the goals that the patient has articulated.

Within a practical policy framework in contrast to theoretical formulations, Brody argues that physicians should not be forced to provide treatment that they believe is futile and inconsistent with professional standards of practice. He argues for futility policies that can be revisited regularly in terms of accumulating scientific data and that include required physician–patient (fam-ily) conversations. He argues that these conversations provide opportunities for full discussion and will lead to informed patient decisions. In most cases, these discussions, which he labels ''autonomy conversations,'' will lead to physician–patient agreement concerning the medical intervention. In those few cases in which there is disagreement and the patient or family insists on a treatment that the physician deems medically futile, one of two conversa-tions should take place. The futility conversation is one in which the physi-cian tries to clarify the reasons why the patient wants the treatment, indicates the professional reasons for denying it, and offers opportunities for consul-tation. The justice conversation is one in which the physician indicates why resource factors preclude provision of the requested treatment.

Both Brody and Norton Spritz (Chapter 4) underscore the importance of separating futility discussions and decisions from those about resource allo-cation or, as such allocation is sometimes called, health care rationing. Al-though arguing for safeguards against physician abuse related to futility judgments and for required physician–patient conversations, Brody provides a consideration of medical futility from a physician-centered perspective. The stakeholders in this discussion, the physicians, have enormous power in mak-ing futility judgments but are equally at risk of being pressured to violate professional standards.

In the midst of what he notes as the ''struggle between physicians and patients for decisional power," Spritz makes a clear case against solutions that favor one or the other of these stakeholders. Rather, he notes an emerging consensus suggesting middle-ground solutions between unlimited patient autonomy and absolute physician empowerment. This consensus involves agreement that unilateral physician futility judgments should be rare and flexibility should be customary. It also involves developing safeguarding mechanisms, such as rigorous adherence to a process to reach institutional agreement rather than relying on having individual physicians label treatments "futile." For example, certain treatments would be classified as futile on the basis of institutional consensus. Patients would be told that institutional policy would permit these treatment choices to be offered only when individually justified. Spritz finds this institutional consensus approach appealing because it removes some of the decisional power, as well as the burdens, from the hands of single physicians and, at least theoretically, permits patients to select institutions with policies that complement their own values and beliefs. However, he also underscores the importance of guidelines and standards for these consensus decisions and strict monitoring.

The issue of medically futile care in the intensive care unit (ICU) is discussed in Chapter 3 by Harry S. Rafkin and Thomas Rainey. These authors cite studies that describe the poor rates of survival to discharge among these desperately ill patients. However, age is not a good predictor of outcome and should not be used as a criterion for assessing the potential benefit of intensive care. ICU patients who have experienced cardiac arrest and received cardiopulmonary resuscitation (CPR) or who have multisystem organ failure have especially low survival rates. Decisions to withdraw or withhold specific therapies and to execute a do not resuscitate (DNR) order must be based on extensive and ongoing discussions with the patient, family, and/or health care proxy (some people prefer the term "health care agent"). The authors quote Quinn's useful definition of futility (Quinn 1994): "treatment [that] cannot within a reasonable probability cure, ameliorate, improve, or restore a quality of life that would be satisfactory to the patient." An advance directive enormously facilitates decisions for patients who lack capacity. The recent SUPPORT study emphasizes the need for patients or their surrogates to voice their wishes strongly (SUPPORT Principal Investigators 1995).

The issues involved in futility judgments about children are vastly more difficult than those relating to adults, particularly the aged. Joel E. Frader and Jon Watchko (Chapter 5) point out that there is universal consensus that the fate of children should be different from that of adults – the intense belief that children should live a natural life span. A further complication is that outcome predictions, particularly for neonates, are much less certain than outcome predictions for adults. Also, unlike the situation with adults, futility decisions for children must be negotiated with surrogates, the parents, and usually nothing is known about what the child might have wanted or chosen.

At the other end of the age spectrum, there are unique aspects to medical futility decisions in nursing home settings. Ellen Bartoldus (Chapter 6) points out that long-term relationships between nursing home staff and patients make it particularly difficult to make and implement decisions that treatment is futile. Staff are attached to patients in powerful ways and resist any actions seen as abandoning them. Bartoldus stresses the importance of helping nursing home staff distinguish between futile medical treatment that should be abandoned and compassionate care that never should be withdrawn or withheld.

Two additional aspects of the nursing home setting differentiate the medical futility debate there from that which takes place in the acute care setting. First, the nature of patient–staff relationships and the duration of stay place the nursing home staff in a particularly good position to help patients understand the importance of clearly stating their treatment preferences. Indeed, staff play a vital role in helping residents think through and reach such decisions. Similarly, nursing home staff are well situated to help residents and their loved ones understand the importance of using advance directives to document end-of-life decisions and to help residents to prepare these documents.

Second, in addition to these educational/counseling roles that nursing home staff play for competent residents and their families, nursing homes provide a unique setting in which to study medical futility decisions related to demented patients. These decisions are particularly challenging when little evidence exists about the subjective experience of the demented patient and, thus, little information about what that patient might want or how he or she might experience the absence of a particular treatment.

Yet another treatment setting deserves consideration. Joseph J. Jacobs (Chapter 7) reports studies with divergent estimates of the use of alternative therapies. Estimates varied from as little as 3% to as much as 66% of the study populations, depending on the diagnoses and demographic variables involved. Thirteen billion dollars of out-of-pocket expenditures represent a conservative estimate of what Americans spend each year on alternative care.

According to Jacobs, the crux of the turn toward nonconventional therapies rests on unwillingness to accept a pessimistic prognosis, defense against the label of ''futile,'' and a profound level of desperation and anxiety that pushes patients to reach out for help from nontraditional sources. The problem, continues Jacobs, in addition to the lack of efficacy or effectiveness data available about alternative therapies, is that patient involvement with such treatments tends to elicit their physicians' frustration and irritation. More exploration of alternative therapies and even more warmth, support, and understanding offered to patients are critical for maintaining a constructive dialogue – the doctor–patient relationship – needed to negotiate the shoals of terminal illness.

Finally, from the physician's side of the equation, James J. Strain, Stephen L. Snyder, and Martin Drooker (Chapter 10) discuss the role of consultation-liaison psychiatrists in helping to resolve conflicts between patients and physicians over futility judgments. Such psychiatrists are particularly adept at assisting patients to shift from their accustomed physical activity to the psychologic activity necessary at the end of life. They also are helpful with families who demand futile treatments because of denial or guilt. C/L psychiatrists have an important role in helping physicians deal with their own maladaptive responses that may result from their intrapersonal issues – overtreating, undertreating, or abandoning patients. Consultation-liaison psychiatrists also assist physicians and other provider staff by interpreting the difficult patients' behavior and words. Strain, Snyder, and Drooker offer remarkably simple but penetrating samples of the questions desperately ill patients ask with words and behavior and of the replies that physicians might make. C/L psychiatrists work with both patients and staff to lessen the conflicts inherent in futility decisions.

Yet another way to accommodate the futility debate and bring some resolution to the disagreements between patients and providers is the use of ethics committees. Alice Herb and Eliot J. Lazar (Chapter 11) describe how institutional ethics committees have become a forum for dispute resolution. The development of ethics committees is based on the prevailing notion that ethical dilemmas should be resolved at the bedside rather than in court. Herb and Lazar point out that although hospital ethics committees are fairly consistently multidisciplinary, including physicians, nurses, social workers, administrators, and frequently bioethics consultants, clergy, attorneys, and community representatives, they vary substantially in sophistication, functions, and acceptance within the institution. Although the amount of attention that ethics committees devote to various functions also differs – education, policy review and development, and case review are among their primary functions – as the committees develop and gain acceptance in their settings, some balance between these functions usually emerges.

In contrast to medical futility seen primarily from the providers' perspective, Patricia Brophy (Chapter 2) offers us a deeply compelling view of the patient/family as stakeholder. Brophy describes her three-year odyssey through the health care and court systems in a frustrating, dehumanizing quest to let her husband die (i.e., withdraw life-sustaining interventions) of catastrophic injuries sustained as a result of a ruptured brain aneurysm and subsequent stroke. Brophy's story abundantly demonstrates the fundamental point that despite years of expert debate about medical futility, society has a long way to go to reach a consensus about acceptable behavior associated with right-to-die matters. Her story demonstrates an often overlooked side to struggles about medical futility: resolution of such struggles must reconcile physical, emotional, psychologic, spiritual, and community considerations.

Although the primary stakeholders in a futility debate are likely to be the physician and patient (family), as the nation reaches an apparent ceiling on resources for health care, society becomes another meaningful stakeholder. Donald J. Murphy (Chapter 12) leads us through a consideration of the economics of futility by noting that the debate is rendered difficult, if not impossible, by the absence of data and consensus about what treatments provided under what circumstances are actually cost effective. In the current environment, relatively few people have advance directives that might limit costly end-of-life treatment or have access to hospice programs that also limit the costs of end-of-life care. Therefore, Murphy suggests that savings may not offset the cost of developing enabling statutes, policies, and procedures to deal with making decisions about medically futile care. Instead, he proposes that the solution rests in expanding the futile intervention debate from one primarily limited to professionals to one that involves the public. Discussing the work of the Colorado Collective for Medical Decisions (CCMD) as an example of how to bring the public constructively into the futility debate, Murphy suggests that futility decisions currently are more about values than economics and that meaningful cost savings would require the country to shift its values from emphasis on individualism to emphasis on communities and resource stewardship.

Cultural and religious attitudes that each of the primary stakeholders bring to the table further confound the debate on both societal and individual levels. Mary F. Morrison and Sarah Gelbach DeMichele (Chapter 8) note that health care professionals frequently have little understanding of their patients' views about health care decision making, life-sustaining technology, and the meaning of life and death, making potentially contentious situations even more so. The authors add that in times of crisis, such as the end of life, individuals' religious and cultural values often are great sources of strength and comfort. Such sources of solace cannot be ignored by providers who may bring different religious and cultural values to discussions with patients.

Morrison and DeMichele briefly review the primary features of a variety of cultural and religious attitudes toward death and end-of-life decision making. However, they note that regardless of the specific values and beliefs, the utmost importance should be attached to having all the stakeholders in the debate clearly state their beliefs so that differences between them can be accommodated. Finally, the authors recognize that although differences may not be resolvable, patients and families nonetheless ''deserve a meaningful and dignified process of death and dying,'' attainable only if cultural and religious factors are clear and taken into consideration.

John J. Paris and Mark Poorman (Chapter 9) extend the discussion with their consideration of the outcomes of conflict between religious beliefs and medical judgments. They present the question raised by Callahan (1994) about whether a good society ''should leave crucial life and death decisions in the hands of individuals or let them be decided, at least in part, by commonly shared, cultural notions of what is and is not'' the appropriate medical response to a dying patient. The authors present the argument that although every individual must be free to hold his or her own values and beliefs, such individual holdings cannot be the basis for public policy. Thus, conflicts that cannot be resolved between patients and their physicians must be settled by establishing public policy and supporting legislation.

Linda Johnson and Robert Lyman Potter (Chapter 14) continue the discussion of community-based efforts to establish medical futility policies by carefully describing a series of projects involving shared decision making at both clinical and societal levels. Rather than shifting the burden of conflict resolution away from the individual practitioner and patient, such programs emphasize community education (Santa Monica/UCLA program), development of consensus among multiple institutions (Minneapolis), efforts to enhance communication among the stakeholders (SUPPORT project), and efforts to produce community consensus about guidelines (Houston, Durham, Sacramento).

Bethany Spielman (Chapter 15) questions the suggestion that the futility debate be taken out of the hands of individual practitioners and patients when the conflict is unresolvable. She contends that institutional, legislative, judicial, and scholarly concern in such weighty matters as medical futility is not unusual but that the extent of community concern now being expressed is surprising and perhaps of limited value.

Spielman indicates that community efforts at developing futility policies stem from a widespread belief that medical futility is a problem of distributive justice that society should be involved in resolving. In addition, health care professionals, disappointed with court findings in many of the futility cases, are looking to other entities, such as communities, as arbiters in the futility debate. These providers also believe that standards of care codified by community policies could be used as a source of evidence for the defense in malpractice suits. Finally, communitarian ethics are experiencing an upsurge in appeal and could be used to moderate the growing tension between patient and physician autonomy.

The problems related to community futility policies reside in their goals. Spielman contends that the proper goal of community efforts should be to provide experiential evidence about which policies work well and which do not and that there should be ongoing evaluation of results attributable to community policies. Improper goals, or at least goals likely to yield substantially diminished returns, are those dedicated to creating new substantive or procedural approaches to dealing with questions about medical futility.

William Prip and Anna Moretti (Chapter 13) point out that the court decision in 1976 that permitted withdrawal of ventilator support from Karen Ann Quinlan provided the impetus for the right-to-die movement. As a result, every state now has laws permitting advance directives, and the federal government has a law that requires health care facilities to inform their patients of their right to execute an advance directive. This landmark decision also focused attention on the right of patients to refuse life-sustaining treatment even when the providers and lawyers wish to continue. The current interest in medical futility has the opposite scenario: physicians wish to discontinue treatment because they have concluded that it has no valid goal, but the patient, or more often the family of a patient who lacks capacity, wishes to continue treatment. These authors quote Meisel, who pointed out that the legal basis for denial of treatment is a well-established negative right that provides the freedom to govern one's own actions unless they interfere with the rights of others. In contrast, the right to receive treatment is not based on a constitutional right, although physicians who deny treatment might be accused of negligence. Prip and Moretti describe the three best-known court cases dealing with medical futility and cite nine others that have some relevance.

These authors suggest that a legal basis for continuing treatment may require action by legislatures rather than the courts. One federal law, the Child Abuse Amendment, and some state laws relating to DNR orders as well as to advance directives now refer specifically to futile treatment. In the case of DNR laws, medical futility is generally taken to mean that the patient will experience repeated arrest in a short time before death occurs. In the case of advance directives, the definition is less clear; treatment is deemed futile if it is medically "inappropriate," "ineffective," "unnecessary," or "contrary to reasonable medical standards."

Risks inherent in the futility debate

The battle for patient autonomy expressed through the right to refuse medical treatment (i.e., have it withdrawn or withheld) was long fought and hard won. This year marks the 20th anniversary of the decision that distinguished the beginning of major progress in this arena.

In contrast, the battle about medical futility has only recently begun in earnest. Questions about when a treatment is futile have not been answered, nor have concerns about who decides these life or death questions been resolved, nor have procedures and processes been developed and tested to address conflicts between the major stakeholders about medical futility decisions. We have yet to reach professional or public consensus even about who the major stakeholders are, much less what each of them brings to the table or needs to take away. Furthermore, although there is an overt problem with medical futility decisions only when there is disagreement among the stakeholders, we have yet to develop and implement systematic ways of looking at the actual decisions and how they are made so that we can determine whether decisions made in the absence of conflict are fair and responsive to the needs of all stakeholders.

Many experts are devoting themselves to finding answers to these questions, and consideration of the future of the medical futility debate would be incomplete without a review of the risks inherent in the emerging approaches to this subject.

Not distinguishing between resource scarcity and medical futility

In the emerging health care delivery environment that is so heavily geared to managed care, there are some subtle and some not so subtle pressures on providers to limit care in order to limit costs. Unless futility decisions can be made in the context of explicit guidelines and criteria, pressures to conserve resources or actual resource scarcity might bias practitioners toward futility decisions that might not be made in the absence of resource constraints. This is a particularly significant risk for vulnerable populations (e.g., poor, elderly, and minority patients). Patients or families of patients from vulnerable groups may respond to subtle, perhaps unconscious, coercion to concur with a futility judgment or simply may not feel able to challenge such decisions.

Safeguards include such strategies as institutional futility policies requiring that futility discussions meet explicit process criteria such as detailed documentation and monitoring and review of decisions against predetermined criteria.

Leaving patients and families out of the decision-making process

The literature suggests that there are clear instances when unilateral decisions about medical futility can and should be made by physicians. Frequently, however, the physicians who make the futility decisions also make the decisions about which stakeholders (e.g., patient, family, consultant, ethics committee) will participate in the decision-making process and when they will do so. In such situations, there is risk that the privilege of unilateral decision making may be abused. Patients and families may be left out of the process even when their inclusion would not necessarily compromise the physicians' decision-making autonomy.

The physician–patient relationship rarely is one in which both parties share the decision-making power equally, and the less powerful participant, the patient, may experience some level of coercion to acquiesce to the other's decisions. This type of pressure may be exacerbated in situations involving not only the patient (family) and physician but also consultants, ethics committees, facility lawyers, and procedural policies established by the facility. This type of pressure also may be exacerbated when the power equation is tipped even further because the patient (family) comes from a vulnerable group, unaccustomed or unfamiliar with ways to challenge the power structure.

Safeguards against this type of risk are twofold. Institutional policies should clearly delineate situations that permit unilateral futility decisions and require that unilateral decisions be documented and prospectively justified. There should be explicit patient (family) representation external to the system (i.e., an unbiased patient advocate) and, again, careful monitoring of the decision making process and review of the decisions.

Shifting futility disagreements to courtrooms, where primacy of the patient is lost

When patient–provider disagreements occur concerning decisions about medical futility, the locus of the ensuing battles may shift away from the bedside into the confrontational atmosphere of the courtroom. There, the focus may shift from the actual needs, well-being, and best interest of the patient to the legal intricacies.

Safeguards include providing a decision-making process, such as external mediation, that focuses on negotiation rather than on confrontation in the event of disagreement.

Shifting the burden of proof inappropriately to patients and families

Institutional policies may establish an unfair burden for patients and their families by creating a list of predetermined conditions considered to be medically futile or, in other ways, make it necessary for patients and their families to demonstrate that their situations are exceptions to the rule. The risk is that in a disagreement about medical futility, patients and families – often without resources and always in crisis – unfairly bear the burden of proving their particular situations to be exceptional.

Safeguards against such risk include providing a predetermined level of assistance to patients and families who are trying to establish their situations as exceptions. In addition, providing accessible explanations of policies before medical futility discussions begin (i.e., before or at admission) also constitutes a safeguard because it allows some measure of freedom for patients to look for a facility that might meet their particular needs. Currently, however, and predictably more so as the managed care system evolves, patient choices about providers are increasingly limited.

Allowing intrapsychic conflicts to influence the way in which power is exerted

As overt struggles between physicians and patients about a variety of issues grow in number and intensity, there is potential for physicians to feel increasingly excluded and for them to try to compensate by making inappropriately unilateral decisions or bringing pressures to bear on patients and families to give informed consent for medical futility decisions.

Once again, *safeguards* involve monitoring decision-making processes when disagreements occur and reviewing ensuing decisions.

Making medical futility decisions based on a clinical bias

Even when decisions about medical futility are made at the bedside rather than in court, there is risk that the patient may get lost in the crisis environment of bedside decision making. When the patient is profoundly ill, the family is distraught, and the physician is under a variety of fiscal and professional pressures, there is risk that decisions about medical futility may emphasize the medical aspects rather than a more complete constellation of factors, including the spiritual, psychologic, and social. There is as yet no clear evidence that cost savings associated with decisions of medical futility would come close to offsetting waste in other areas of the health care system. Without such evidence, some of the decisions to forgo treatment made with a clear clinical bias may be unnecessary.

Safeguards include rigorously applied and monitored requirements that decisions about medical futility consider psychosocial factors. Perhaps an even better safeguard involves moving at least part of the decision-making process to an earlier point. If physicians, patients, and families discuss the patient's values and beliefs about death and end-of-life care, there is a record, hopefully on paper, that provides valuable data to feed into the decision-making process. These data are far more difficult to obtain in a crisis situation than in a more relaxed, nonadversarial clinical setting, such as during an annual physical examination or outpatient treatment visit.

In summary, if the risks inherent in our evolving approaches to making decisions about medical futility are unrecognized or not dealt with, they may seriously compromise the accuracy and fairness of decisions. However, by building a variety of safeguards into the decision-making process, decisions can be protected from the risks discussed here.

Scenarios and solutions: a look to the future

More data will be gathered

Judgments about medical futility often become contentious because they frequently must be made in the absence of good data about likely outcomes of treatment or nontreatment. More empirical data should be gathered, and the rationale and criteria underlying judgments about medical futility should continue to be revisited on an ongoing basis.

The focus of the decision making process will shift

Currently, decisions about medical futility are made in a crisis environment at the bedside of desperately ill patients, frequently without knowledge about the patients' values and beliefs. Patients and their families are anxious and lack the knowledge and experience needed to challenge decisions made in an overwhelmingly clinical atmosphere. It is likely, however, that as more attention is paid to the decision-making process and it is codified in more formal ways, a patient advocacy component will be included. Thus, the process of making decisions about futility will shift from being a primarily physician-centered activity to one that is at least somewhat more patient centered. We may move from talking about medical futility to decisions about patient-appropriate care.

In addition, the decision-making process will shift to an earlier time, when it is easier to lay the groundwork for mutually acceptable decisions. Hopefully, this will reduce the number of serious conflicts and the tendency to resolve those conflicts in court rather than in the clinical setting.

The concept, practice, and availability of palliative care will grow substantially

A movement is growing in this country to refocus end-of-life treatment away from interventions designed to eliminate or slow the disease process to interventions designed to treat symptoms and make patients as comfortable as possible. Experts involved in the movement toward more and improved palliative care stress eloquently that something always can and should be done for the patient and are moving away from current medical perceptions that palliative care is less worthy care and represents giving up. Emphasizing patient-appropriate care in contrast to medical futility will bring the debate's abstract theories closer to practical actions and, thus, will bring providers and patients closer together to solve end-of-life treatment dilemmas constructively.

Educational interventions will increase dramatically

Efforts to teach the public how to think about end-of-life treatment and to make decisions about such treatment are well underway. Currently, there is increasing emphasis on facilitating early patient discussion with families and providers about cultural and spiritual attitudes and beliefs about care at the end of life. Once patients become more vocal about such matters in their interactions with health care providers, patients and their providers, together, will have more information on which to base better decisions.

Physicians also are beginning to receive better training about end-of-life matters. Significant programs are developing to improve training for new physicians about care of the dying patient and to provide better continuing education for practicing physicians in the same arena. Efforts also are beginning to improve the image of end-of-life care so that physicians are more likely to learn, practice, and receive gratification from providing such care.

There will be more formal and explicit policies and procedures for making end-of-life treatment decisions, including those concerning medical futility

Such policies and procedures, as well as rigorously applied monitoring and review systems, will accomplish much in educating patients about the rationale for decisions and their role in the process and will also provide an impetus and support for better decision making by physicians.

Conclusion

Current and emerging philosophy and practice about care at the end of life suggest that we will move away from a concept of purely medical futility to provision of patient-appropriate care based on decisions that patients, families, and physicians reach together. Palliative care will be considered an important medical intervention and will be provided as aggressively and actively as high-technology therapeutic interventions are provided now. All of this is based, after all, on a concept articulated in 1927: "The secret of the care of the patient is in caring for the patient" (Peabody 1927). Thus, this comprehensive consideration of medical futility will become the next to the last word.

References

Callahan, D. 1994. Necessity, futility, and the good society. *Journal of the American Geriatrics Society* 42:866–7.

Fins, J.J., ed. 1994. Futility in clinical practice: report on a congress of clinical societies. *Journal of the American Geriatrics Society* 42:861–905.

Peabody, F.W. 1927. The care of the patient. *Journal of the American Medical Association* 88:877–82. *Cited in* Keyhole, D. 1995. Dancing across the lines: people in pain. *Palliative Care* 11:26–9.

Pearlman, R.A. 1994. Medical futility: where do we go from here? *Journal of the American Geriatrics Society* 42:904–5.

Quinn, J.B. 1994. Taking back their health care. *Newsweek* June 27, p. 36.

SUPPORT Principal Investigators. 1995. A controlled trial to improve care for seriously ill hospitalized patients. The Study to Understand Prognoses and Preferences for Outcomes and Risks of Treatment (SUPPORT). *Journal of the American Medical Association* 274:1591–8.

Index of cited authors, cases, and statutes

Note: The page number on which the reference appears is italicized.

193

Subject index

198